WHO
NEEDS
FRIENDS

Also by Andrew McCarthy

The Longest Way Home

Just Fly Away

Brat

Walking with Sam

WHO NEEDS FRIENDS

AN UNSCIENTIFIC EXAMINATION OF MALE FRIENDSHIP ACROSS AMERICA

ANDREW McCARTHY

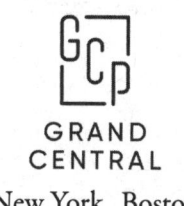

GRAND CENTRAL

New York Boston

In several cases, the names of men I spoke with have been changed—either to protect privacy or to avoid potentially confusing repetition. In two instances, the locations of the conversations have been altered for clarity of storytelling.

Copyright © 2026 by Andrew McCarthy

Jacket design by Elizabeth Connor. Jacket photo courtesy of the author.
Jacket copyright © 2026 by Hachette Book Group, Inc.

Hachette Book Group supports the right to free expression and the value of copyright. The purpose of copyright is to encourage writers and artists to produce the creative works that enrich our culture.

The scanning, uploading, and distribution of this book without permission is a theft of the author's intellectual property. If you would like permission to use material from the book (other than for review purposes), please contact permissions@hbgusa.com. Thank you for your support of the author's rights.

Grand Central Publishing
Hachette Book Group
1290 Avenue of the Americas, New York, NY 10104
grandcentralpublishing.com
@grandcentralpub

First Edition: March 2026

Grand Central Publishing is a division of Hachette Book Group, Inc.
The Grand Central Publishing name and logo is a registered trademark of Hachette Book Group, Inc.

The publisher is not responsible for websites (or their content) that are not owned by the publisher.

Grand Central Publishing books may be purchased in bulk for business, educational, or promotional use. For information, please contact your local bookseller or the Hachette Book Group Special Markets Department at special.markets@hbgusa.com.

Map by Julia Raketic/Shutterstock.com
Print book interior design and map detailing by Bart Dawson

Library of Congress Control Number: 2025948585

ISBNs: 9781538768945 (hardcover), 9781538781371 (hardcover signed edition), 9781538768969 (ebook)

Printed in the United States of America

LSC-C

Printing 1, 2026

For my friends

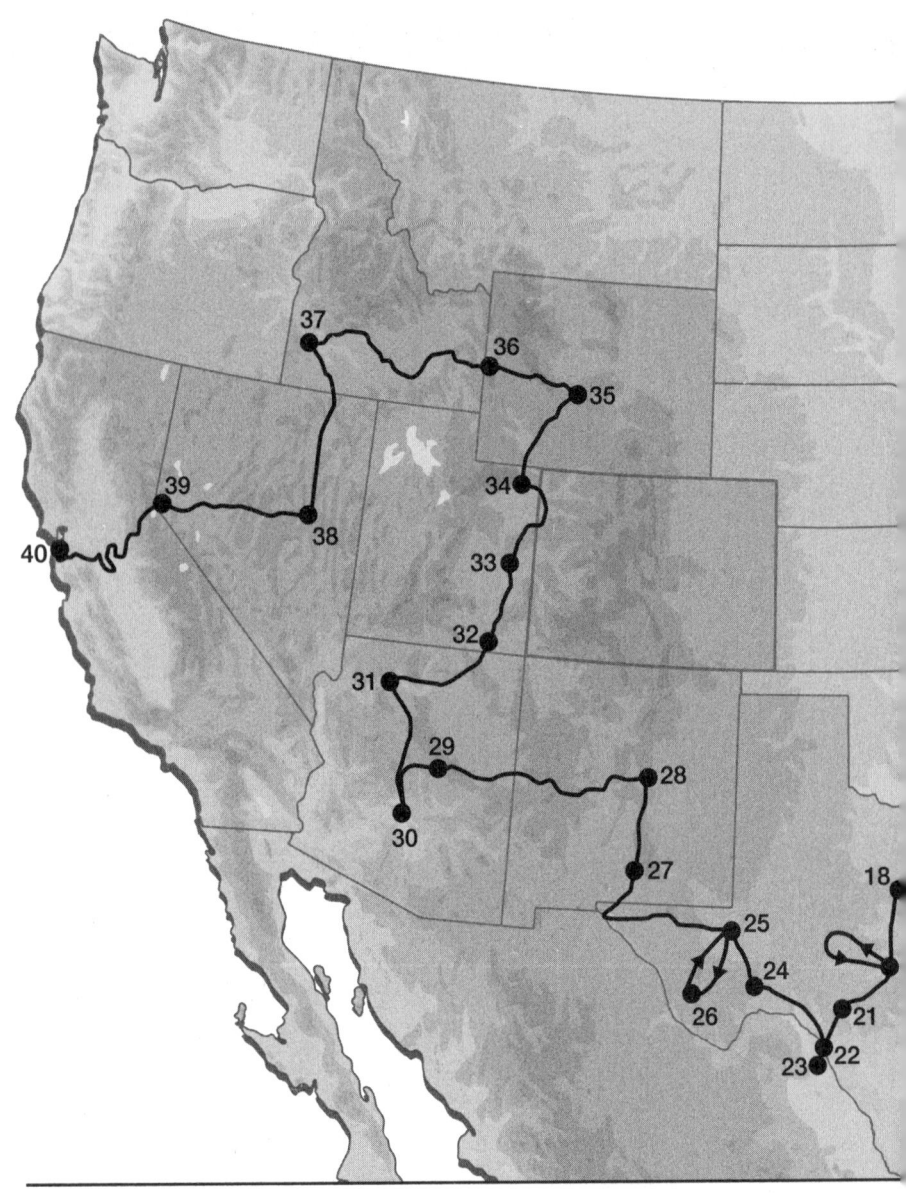

1. New York, NY
2. Atlantic City, NJ
3. Baltimore, MD
4. Philadelphia, PA
5. Harpers Ferry, WV
6. Elkins, WV
7. Point Pleasant, WV
8. Brookville, OH
9. Paris, KY
10. Lexington, KY
11. Leipers Fork, TN
12. Tupelo, MS
13. Oxford, MS
14. Money, MS
15. Clarksdale, MS
16. Natchez, MS
17. Natchitoches, LA
18. Cleburne, TX
19. Shreveport, LA
20. Austin, TX
21. Uvalde, TX

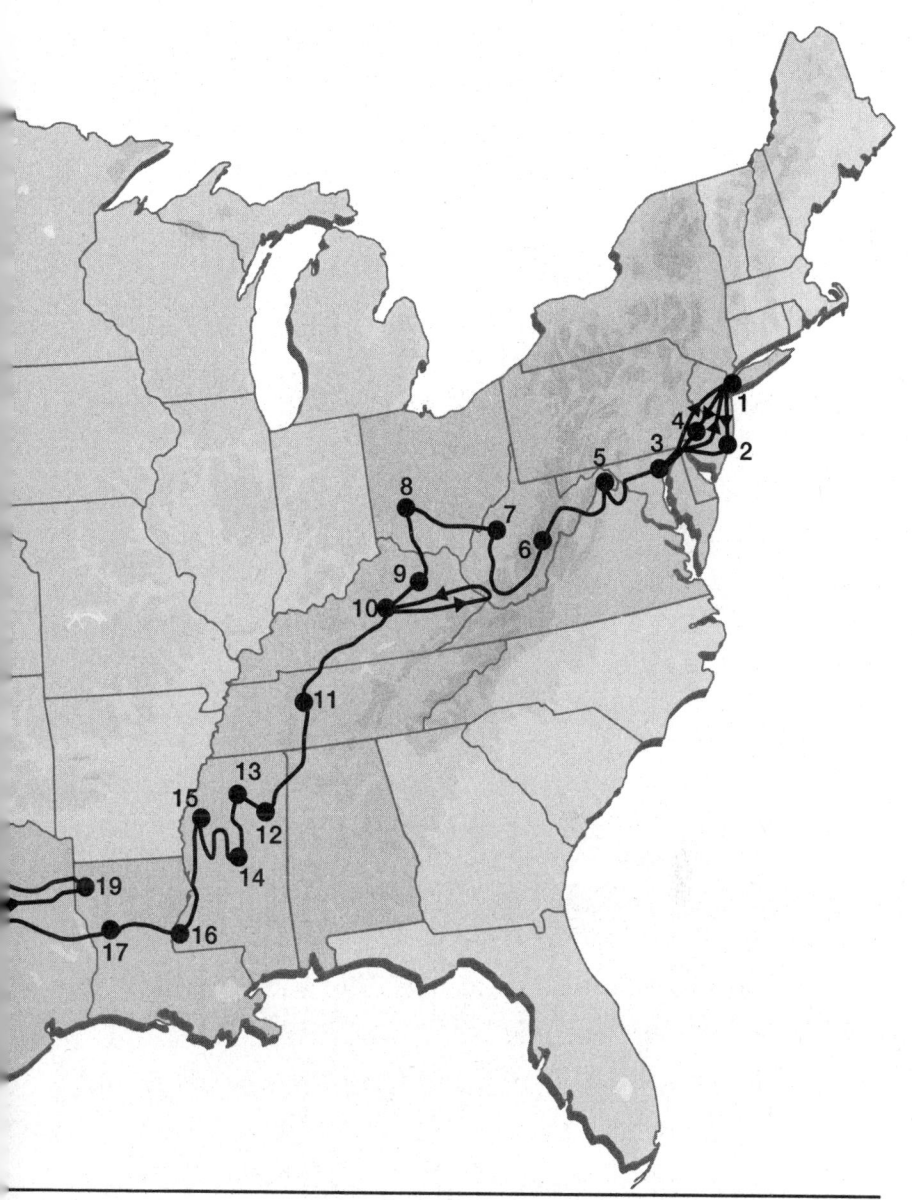

22. Eagle Pass, TX
23. Piedras Negras, Mexico
24. Comstock, TX
25. Wink, TX
26. Marfa, TX
27. White Sands, NM
28. Sandia Park, NM
29. Winslow, AZ
30. Sedona, AZ
31. Grand Canyon, AZ
32. Monument Valley, UT
33. Moab, UT
34. Vernal, UT
35. Lander, WY
36. Jackson Hole, WY
37. Boise, ID
38. Eureka, NV
39. Lake Tahoe, CA
40. Berkeley, CA

WHO
NEEDS
FRIENDS

Lake Tahoe, California

There's a strong smell of pine. A thin band of golden light clings to the horizon above the jagged peaks of the Sierra Nevada Mountains to the west. Overhead, the sky is already a deep blue, almost purple. The first stars are visible.

The glass doors of the nearby hotel bar are thrown open, in defiance of the end of the season—the band is playing a Fleetwood Mac cover that carries the inside outside. A few people are down on the beach beside the marina taking photos. Almost all the boats are already out of the water. I snap a photo of the people snapping photos in the dying light and go around to find the gelato shop.

It isn't an impressive place, containing a lone freezer offering up eight flavors. There are a few metal tables scattered around. The chairs have those wire backs twisted into heart shapes. There's also a fenced-in patio with plastic flowers stuck into pots beside a few more tables and heart-backed chairs. Other than the teenage girl behind the counter, the shop is deserted. And despite the name of the place claiming otherwise, the gelato isn't really even gelato. It's more of a hard ice cream. It doesn't matter.

I chose this spot because it offered me a twenty-minute walk after dinner and then a twenty-minute walk back to my hotel. I just needed to move my body. I've been in the car most of the day—as I have been for weeks and weeks.

I take a seat on one of the heart-backed chairs. It won't rest flat on the ground and I tip back and forth between front right and back left legs while eating my hazelnut ice cream and considering a second scoop. The bored teenage girl who served me comes out from behind the counter. She carelessly swipes the cloth in her hand across an already clean table and asks where I'm from.

"New York," I tell her.

"Whoa," she says. "What are you doing in Tahoe?"

"Passing through. I've been traveling to see my friends."

"That's cool," she says, pushing a stray strand of blond hair back behind her ear. She's maybe seventeen and has one arm in a sling. Her name is Sarah. She's a local girl.

"What happened to your arm, Sarah?"

"I was on my friend's shoulders, and he dropped me." Sarah rolls her eyes. "He was drunk."

"Friends." I shrug.

"Yeah," she says. "You drive the whole way?"

I nod.

"Where else you been?"

"Oh, um," I begin, almost embarrassed, "I've been through twenty-two states, so…"

"Really?"

"I didn't plan it that way. It just sort of happened."

"How many miles is that?"

"About ten thousand."

"Ten thousand?" Sarah sounds incredulous. "How does driving ten thousand miles just sort of happen?"

I try to laugh. "Especially since I hate driving."

Sarah shakes her head at my seeming folly.

"Not very smart, is it?" I say.

"Not unless you have a good reason."

"I do," I say. And anyway, I'm almost there. Tomorrow night I'll be at the Pacific, having dinner with my friend.

I explain to Sarah that besides reuniting with my friends, I've also been talking to other men—cowboys and retired cops, blues musicians and oil rig workers, journalists, recovering junkies, former military, preachers, rootless teens—talking with them about their experience with friendship.

"Really?" Sarah says, simultaneously confused and curious.

"Yeah. It's been surprising," I say to Sarah. "And it turns out that a lot of guys have a difficult time with friendship."

Sarah sinks into one hip and looks at me like I'm an idiot. "Yeah," she says. "No kidding."

New York, New York

I was seated at the kitchen table drinking a cup of weak tea. The dog was asleep in the corner. My twenty-one-year-old son sat cross-legged on the floor, messing with his electric guitar, telling me a funny story about a dating disaster involving one of his good friends.

"Rocco's a fool," I said with affection when Sam's tale was done.

"He is," Sam agreed. "I love him."

We laughed. Then Sam stopped strumming and looked at me. "You don't really have any friends, do you, Dad?"

The directness of my son's comment was typical of him, but Sam didn't mean it in a hurtful or aggressive way. As far as he knew, it was a fair enough assessment. But as is the case between parents and their children, there's more to the story of my life than my son is aware. I looked at him.

"I have friends, Sam," I said. "I just don't see them, but I know they're there. And that's enough."

Somewhere I must have known that Sam had hit a nerve, because I instantaneously and unconsciously adopted an attitude that spoke from a parental height. My tone was infused with wisdom and understanding, and allowed me to share my insight with my son in a spirit of openness and generosity.

Sam considered me—probably knew I was full of shit (even if I didn't at the moment)—then graciously accepted my answer with a brief nod. We chatted some more, and he went off to meet his girlfriend.

His comment stayed with me.

What had actually happened to my friendships? Were they still there, as I claimed? Did I even want them? Or need them? What did I get from them, anyway? What did I have to offer them? How did friendship affect my place in the world? What did I value? What mattered?

I sipped my tea—it was cold. My eighteen-year-old daughter, Willow, raced through, late for a dance class. The dog lifted her head at this excitement, stretched, then went back to sleep.

My experience with friendship has not always been straightforward.

Growing up in suburban New Jersey, mine was a typical neighborhood upbringing, now long gone—driveway basketball games and stolen peeks at *Playboy* magazine in wood-paneled basements. "Be home at six for dinner" was my mother's after-school mantra. I was the third of four boys. My older brother Peter was my protector. I was a shy kid with a small circle, yet never wanted for friends.

In my early twenties I became successful in the movies. "Overnight," my position in the world was forever altered. I was a very unprepared public figure. Someone who was content to slip along the edges, desiring to be special yet not craving overt attention, I was thrust into the center of things. People came at me. I wrapped myself tighter around the friends I had before this burst of notoriety. That I began to drink too much spoke to my innate alcoholism and not to my newfound fortune.

I retreated, then withdrew.

By the time this brush with fame had subsided and my drinking had been arrested, I was nearly thirty, and a more solitary version of who I was began to emerge. I discovered I liked my own company and often sought out time alone.

When eventually I married, I saw that almost all my friendships with women had been based around flirtation and the possibility of our going to bed. That obviously had to change. And with men, I looked up to realize that my several close and longtime friends had moved away. Far away.

On the rare occasion I did form a new connection, the motivation to nurture it was often lacking. Whether a reaction to the hollowness of some insincere friendships made during my early fame, or a fearful nature, or just becoming set in my habits, I found myself uninterested, even unwilling, to reach out to new friends. No matter—I was happy in my own company and with that of my wife and children. And there was always work. Life felt full—at least full enough.

But sitting alone at the kitchen table, dog asleep in the corner, my now-cold tea in hand, I became aware that this was one of those moments that occasionally present themselves and, by the very nature of its almost imperceptible arrival, demand a reckoning.

Something my wife had cautioned me against came back to me—my introspection, my introversion, my avoidance, had begun to chip away at the edges of who I was and narrow my experience, diminish my joy, limit what I had to offer and what I allowed myself to receive. Rather than relax into an uncomplicated enjoyment of others, expand into an attitude of increased curiosity and easily offered generosity that age might ideally encourage, intermittent bouts of bitterness now had to be fought back. Silent disappointments became normalized. My kids had affectionately (?) begun to accuse me of becoming a curmudgeon. If I was really willing to look, the answer was there to see—my self-induced isolation was diminishing my life, making me into a smaller man.

At one point my friends had been instrumental in broadening my horizons, bolstering my courage, providing safe harbor. But were my dearest friendships—as Sam's question suggested—even still there? There was Seve, a surrogate big brother I met when I was barely twenty. Matthew, a show business confidant I met just a few years later. Eddie, my oldest friend and early role model. And there were two men I'd met in more recent years, John and Don. Dear friends all.

In many ways they were the cornerstones on which so much of my life had been built. I couldn't remember the last time I'd seen any of them. On the rare occasions when I spoke with one of these men on the phone, there were easy laughs and some catching up, but was that just the fumes of past glories?

My solo habits had drawn me into a tightening spiral. Could my friends throw me a line and help pull me from my self-willed exile?

My son's offhand comment had jolted me and yanked down the curtain I had drawn in front of me.

I needed to see my friends.

I picked up my phone. For no reason other than that he was my oldest friend, I called Eddie first. I suggested flying down to Texas for a visit. "For sure," he said. "We should even take some kind of a road trip, to Vegas or Tahoe or someplace." Eddie loved a good road trip, especially if it ended at a casino. "But I gotta finish this fucking building first." Eddie bought and renovated old buildings for a living and was in the middle of a large new project. "Just give me a few months."

I reached out to Matthew. He was quick to say yes to my coming down to Kentucky. I bought a plane ticket. Then, days before my flight, he called to cancel. "There's just too much shit going on," Matthew said. "Work is a mess, and Ev (his son Everett) is in the middle of some stuff." Perhaps I knew something like this might happen because I had bought a refundable plane ticket—something I never did. We pushed it a few weeks, and I rescheduled my flight. Then he canceled again. "Let's just do it in the spring," Matthew said decisively. "Things should calm down by then." I refunded my plane ticket.

John was mountain climbing in the Himalayas. Don's email autoreply said that he was in Japan for an extended stay.

When Seve and I finally connected, he was excited by the idea and also suggested we hit the road—"I've wanted to head down to the Chesapeake Bay," Seve said. "It's just a couple days, but that's probably all my back can take." My friend had developed terrible back trouble. Several years ago, he underwent a major operation to address stenosis, a narrowing of the spine. Nerves were being pinched, and the pain had become intolerable. The recovery was long and arduous. I wasn't there to help or even visit. More important, the operation hadn't done the trick; his back was worse than ever. Another operation was being recommended. This one would require him to be on the table for eight hours.

I was eager to reconnect.

Then the day before I was headed down to Baltimore, my friend called to cancel, citing a doctor's appointment. It seemed odd that he didn't know about the conflict in advance, but I let it pass. We rescheduled. Then, a few weeks later, just as I was walking out the door to see him, my phone rang again.

"I haven't been entirely honest with you," Seve began, the strain in his voice palpable.

"Okay," I said, suddenly aware to keep my tone neutral.

"I'm not in great shape. I can't really walk very far, and sitting in a car for that long would be brutal on my back."

"That's fine. We don't need to go far."

"And I'm up and down all night long. My sleep schedule is all turned around. It's not the right time. Let's just postpone it a little."

"All right," I said reluctantly. "Why don't I just come down and take you to dinner."

"I don't want you to drive all that way."

"I was gonna do that anyway," I assured him. "It's a few hours. It's nothing."

"I'm just really not up for it. I really appreciate it, but please hear me." My friend was imploring me now. "It is not a good time. We'll do it soon. I promise."

I could hear the pain, even fear, in Seve's voice now. "Okay, Seve," I said. "No sweat. We'll do it soon."

I hung up, glanced at my overnight bag by the door, made a cup of weak tea, and took a seat in my customary spot at the kitchen table. The dog came over and nudged me for a pet. I shooed her away.

It was natural that my friends had full and busy lives. While disappointed, I took no offense. I understood—or so I told myself.

And then the longer I sat with that phone call from Seve, the less comfortable I felt about it. My friend sounded in trouble. I had not been there for our relationship for too long. Was it too late? Had I let the friendship atrophy too much? Was it now just going to fade away entirely? Was I being too melodramatic to think that I didn't want the next time I saw my friend to be at his funeral?

That night I couldn't sleep. The pain I heard in Seve's voice—I kept replaying the conversation.

I got in the car.

Seve

Atlantic City, New Jersey

I don't remember the first time I met Seve. I do know that I was living on the top floor of a six-story walk-up on Bank Street in Greenwich Village in Manhattan. Eddie had gone off on what was supposed to be a six-month trip around the world (he made it as far as Thailand and stayed) and had ensconced me in his apartment. I was a nineteen-year-old kid. My next-door neighbor, Nita, was a grown woman in her late twenties. We had an open-door policy, meaning that Nita could come into my apartment whenever she wanted, while I was free to knock on her door. And one day I met her boyfriend, Seve.

(It should be noted that Seve's actual name is not Seve, but Stephen. Years ago, our mutual friend Eddie ironically dubbed Stephen Seve, in reference to the beloved, swashbuckling Spanish golfer, Seve Ballesteros. Stephen, for all his athletic ability, lacked any grace on the golf course. I have not called Seve Stephen in nearly forty years).

Unlike his girlfriend, and even though he was a decade older than me, Seve regarded me as an equal. As a young person anxious to be viewed as an adult in the world, this endeared him to me instantly. We began to play tennis together. We'd sometimes grab a burger at the Corner Bistro down the street. On Sunday afternoons we'd often talk on the phone, *New York Times* travel section on our laps, and plot where we ought to visit someday. Then on a cold Christmas Day I called him up and suggested we get in a taxi, drive to the airport, and actually go somewhere.

"When, now?" Seve asked.

"Now," I said.

Seve surprised me by picking me up in a cab a half hour later. Soon we were looking up at the departures board at Newark Airport. People's Express—one of the original and most cut-rate of the cut-rate airlines—had a flight to Puerto Rico leaving in an hour. We bought two tickets. That night we were in a bar in San Juan. A man with a Hemingway beard who spoke English with a Spanish accent sat on the stool beside us. He whispered of an island just off the coast—Vieques. A paradise, he said. The navy frequently shelled the tiny isle for target practice, but we shouldn't worry about such things, the artillery was well aimed, and besides, it was Christmas, surely the navy would be on a break from the bombing.

We lay in our beds that night and made a mental list of all the things we would need to bring to our primitive paradise. The next morning, we boarded a six-seater plane for the twenty-minute flight. The arrivals terminal was an eight-by-twelve, three-sided cinder block shed with a corrugated metal roof containing a tiny desk beside a large scale and a small bar with three stools. It also doubled as the departures terminal.

A young, effete man with minimal English came by and gestured for us to follow him on foot. He knew a place to stay. The roads were sand or ruptured pavement (torn up from the shelling?). The foliage was scraggly and unkempt. We saw no cars and no people. Such simplicity would be my idea of heaven today, but as a young man, mai tais and swimming pools were more my notion of paradise. My spirits were falling fast. Our escort led us to what he said was the one hotel on the island. A trim man with a mustache behind the reception desk offered us a confidential smile. "We're glad you're here," he purred. Seve and I had a look around. The place was as ragtag as everything else. There were several clusters of men lounging around looking like they had been doped. Seve leaned over to me. "There are no women here," he said. Women or no women, I told Seve I was returning to the airport.

Back at the cinder block shed/departures lounge we learned the only flight of the day didn't leave for another six hours. I asked what was in the blue cooler behind the bar. Beer. We pulled up two stools. By the time our flight was to board (Seve and I were its only two passengers), we were well oiled, and I think we both regretted leaving.

The other seats on the tiny plane were crammed with crates and boxes, and the pilot turned to us. "Would you mind if I stop at St. Thomas on the way to drop some things? It'll save me a trip."

"I didn't like San Juan anyway," I said, and we got off with the cargo.

A dreadlocked Rastafarian was behind the wheel of a cab idling under a tree at the St. Thomas airport. We climbed in the back. "How you doing?" Seve asked.

"Cool and quiet, mon, cool and quiet" came the languid reply.

He knew a hotel, he said, and while en route I asked, "Anywhere we can get some ganja?"

The driver shifted his bloodshot eyes to me in the rearview mirror and made the next left.

"My cousin's place," he said as we pulled up in front of a small bar with Jimmy Cliff blaring through the walls. The only two non-Rastafarians in the shack, Seve and I were high from second-hand smoke before we ever met the "cousin."

Properly stoned, we were deposited at a hotel (with pool) on a hilltop.

"This is more like it," I said to my friend.

In the middle of the night I woke, itching. I could hear Seve tossing in the other bed. "Fuck," he shouted. Then came the slap of flesh. "There are bedbugs in here!"

We went out to sit by the swimming pool. The air was close. There were no stars. The only light came from the still illuminated (but unheated) pool. Bathed in an aqua-blue cast, we sat.

"I wish I hadn't answered the phone when you called," my friend said.

"You don't mean that, Seve."

He grumbled.

"Well," I said, trying to look on the bright side, "at least it's not raining."

Lightning flashed. It began to rain.

Hard.

And we started to laugh.

It was the kind of hysterical laughter over which a lifelong friendship is forged.

As my brother Peter and I drifted apart through the strains of geography and divergent lives, Seve in many ways became my surrogate big brother. When I started to get successful in the movies, Seve grew protective. Where other people came at me wanting, Seve put his arm around my shoulder. Decades before personal branding was an ideal, Seve urged me to think of myself as a commodity and to strategize. I was too young and felt too precarious about my prospects to act on or even understand his advice. Seve spoke truth to me, and for my part, I spoke it back—not because I felt any strong belief in my opinions, but because in many ways I felt that my words carried such little weight, had so little consequence, that I could speak them readily.

Over the next decade, as I grew up and grew in confidence, Seve and I continued to travel together, and we grew closer. He would visit if I was working—in London, Paris, Spain, Scotland. We took several long and memorable road trips through Ireland, drinking, golfing, getting lost. We drove across the country together from LA to NY.

Seve's work often took him away. A born salesman, he was a road warrior, handling strategic planning and the marketing of dental products for several large companies. Because he loved motivating people, saw beyond their weaknesses and highlighted their strengths, he inspired loyalty and made interesting what sounded to me like inherently boring work.

When I began to write about travel, Seve joined me on several of my early assignments. Never more himself than when offering up support, Seve was a natural cheerleader and coach. I felt emboldened on the road with Seve by my side. For his part, Seve delighted in my impulsiveness. Although we never discussed it, I knew he took pride in our friendship. It brought us both joy.

And Seve was there when I met my second wife in the west of Ireland. "That's lightning," he cautioned me when he first saw Dolores and me together. Seve was my best man at my wedding with Dolores in Dublin.

Work eventually forced Seve to relocate, first to LA (where I still saw him often, since I was frequently there for my own work) then to Denver, and finally back to Baltimore, where he was born. Other than the occasional mention of playing sports in school, and the one time I met his sister and mother for pizza, Seve rarely focused on or filled me in about the story of his youth. So I was surprised one day while visiting him in Baltimore when he drove me out to show me where he grew up.

It was a two-story, redbrick building, part of a lower middle-class suburban apartment complex in a modest neighborhood, across the street from an unkempt field. The humility of the place surprised me. Without realizing it, I had imagined that Seve grew up much as I had in New Jersey, in a more upscale middle-class suburban neighborhood of pleasant houses and tidy lawns. We parked and looked over at the apartment building.

"Those windows on the second floor, that was us," Seve said, almost in bewilderment.

"Let's go look," I said, and got out of the car.

"Wait," Seve called, trying to stop me.

We crossed the street and approached the building. There was no lock on the front door. I followed Seve up a flight of stairs to a small landing with two opposing doors. He turned to the one on the left.

"This was it," Seve said.

We stood in silence, and I watched my friend look at the white door, his expression inscrutable. After a long while he chuckled softly, in the "life is crazy" way that I've seen Seve do often, and we returned to the car.

"Thanks, Seve," I said after I closed the door.

He looked past me and nodded toward the scraggly field. "I was in that park every day," he said softly. And we drove away.

As my family grew, my time felt more constrained. I took solace in knowing that Seve was out there, but it didn't make up for getting together; if anything, it helped diffuse the urgency to do so. We'd still talk on the phone, but that too seemed to happen with less and less frequency. When we did connect it was—as close friends often say—like no time had passed. And if life for now was calling the shots, we could at least talk about getting together "someday."

But now that "someday" is today.

At nine thirty on a Thursday morning in late September, I walk out of my Manhattan apartment, get in my car, drive west on Seventy-Seventh Street, turn downtown on West End Avenue, pass the car dealerships, and squeeze into the Lincoln Tunnel. Emerging into the muted light of New Jersey, I'm deposited onto the turnpike—the road named by the *Huffington Post* as one of "The Top Ten Absolute Worst Places to Drive in the World."

In my eagerness to see Seve, I've left far too early. My friend—whose movements have been largely restricted due to his bad back—has apparently become a night owl, often sleeping the days away while drifting through the wee, wee hours. So, with time to kill, I'm considering a side trip into our mutual past. On our initial call Seve talked about returning to Atlantic City—so that's where I head first.

Beyond the Exxon Bayway refinery in Linden, I merge onto the Garden State Parkway, and in a few hours, I'm swerving onto the Atlantic City Expressway, past the boarded-up American Star Inn, the deserted Journeys End motel, the dilapidated Goodfellas Pub. A dead raccoon lies by the side of the road. At the causeway over the swamp that separates Atlantic City from the mainland, a billboard boasts a Stevie Nicks concert that took place seven months earlier. Three large wind turbines struggle to turn—they weren't there the last time I came this way, decades earlier with Seve and Eddie.

Things downtown are not much more hopeful. Running parallel to the Atlantic Ocean is Pacific Avenue. Howard Johnson's advertises a midweek special of free internet. Across from the Hard Rock Hotel and Casino, Rosa D'Oro promises "CA$H for your gold." No one is on the street.

In the garage at Caesars, I have my pick of spots to park, then make my way through the ghostly casino to the boardwalk. The Atlantic rolls into a long and deserted beach, save for a lone man sweeping a metal detector back and forth over the gray sand. The sun is a vague orb behind a thick bank of clouds. Across from the shuttered miniature golf course is Atlantic City's convention hall, where a plaque boasts that in 1977 Governor Brendan T. Byrne signed the Casino Control Act, enabling New Jersey to become only the second state to allow gambling. The detritus of what followed surrounds me.

A small, wiry man, a victim of his own nervous energy, in a bright yellow shirt embroidered with the words "Visitor Services" over the breast pocket, approaches me like a buzzing bee. "That there is where the Trump Plaza used to be." He points behind me to an empty, weed-filled lot I hadn't been considering, shaking his small head. "He's long gone."

Kenny, a local born and bred, is an "ambassador" for the city.

"What do you do as an ambassador, Kenny?"

"Just this. Make everyone feel welcome. Keep things moving."

Then the ambassador, with his arms waving about, surprises me with his frankness. "I'll tell you this much, this town is going under. Another ten years and it'll all be over."

"Really?" I say just to say something.

"Oh, yeah. I'm sixty-three years old, so I can remember when Atlantic City was Atlantic City."

"When was that?" I ask.

"The seventies, eighties."

"I came here in the eighties with my friends," I say. Seve, Eddie, and I made impulsive and not infrequent late-night runs down to Atlantic City—ill-advised decisions fueled by youthful stupidity and alcohol.

"Really?" Kenny says, eager that I perhaps share his recollections of those heady days.

"Oh, yeah," I say, "the place used to jump."

"Jump? Man, we was on fire in the eighties. But that's all finished now. This town is over. Everyone's moved away, 'cept me."

"You still got some friends here?"

"Friends? Man, I got so many friends, I don't know what to do with 'em all." Then Kenny stops twitching and his shoulders and arms slump, like a marionette whose strings have been dropped. "But they all gone now," he confesses. "Moved away or gone. It's Lonelyville now."

An autumn wind blows in off the ocean, and Kenny rallies. "But I got me a nice room. Got a good window and a comfy chair. So, I'm good. But yeah, it's all over. You know what I'm saying?"

"I do," I say, stifling the urge to explain to Kenny that this is exactly what I'm doing on the road and why I've returned here, to this place my friends and I, in our innocence, used to frequent, a place where we felt so alive, so invincible, so bonded to one another. It was a time when the future was friendly, everything felt possible. And I don't want it to be, as Kenny says, "all over."

Back through the cavernous casino, waiting at the elevator, a song catches my attention and sounds like it's being sung directly to me. I lift my iPhone and ask Siri what's playing. The tune in question is titled "In a Little While."

...I feel like something is gone here... the singer laments. Then another line jumps out—*...I've lost what I'd found.*

Feeling exhausted now, my limbs heavy, I make my way through the deserted parking garage, relieved to find that no one's broken into my car.

Baltimore, Maryland

I'm still a few hours from Baltimore. On the way out of Atlantic City, just past the American Way Check Cashing shop, a billboard reminds me that Christ died for my sins. A right turn puts me onto US Route 40.

You'd be hard-pressed to imagine it now, but from this inauspicious corner, US Route 40 once stretched the length of the country to San Francisco 3,157 miles to the west. Known as "The Main Street of America," it was a major artery across the nation. But with the advent of the Interstate Highway System in the 1950s, the road lost its relevancy. It terminates now near Salt Lake City, Utah, and while still a fair drive from the Jersey shore, the glory days of US 40—like those of Atlantic City—are, as Kenny lamented, "all over."

Strip malls, a tuxedo rental shop, a mortuary, then scraggly scrub. Away from the coast the terrain becomes a more rural type of suburbia. No sidewalks line unmanicured streets. Patches of farmland appear.

At the Delaware River I'm funneled back onto the strain of I-95. Two Hyundais race past at high speed on either side. One swerves in front of me to cut the other off in a game of high-stakes chicken. Red taillights flare. I look where I can take up Route 40 again. But there's little relief as 40 has become eight lanes of stop-and-go lined with Taco Bells, power lines, traffic signals.

A giant rooftop sign proclaims "GUNS." After almost being T-boned by a massive SUV running a red light, I say, "Fuck it," to the empty car and get back on I-95 all the way to Baltimore.

A few quick turns off the interstate and I'm in the parking lot outside Seve's condo. It's nearly empty. The marina he lives on in Baltimore's Outer Harbor is purportedly under renovation, although there's no evidence that work has begun. Disoriented and stiff after the drive, I wander around the building looking for an entrance. It's late in the afternoon now, the day growing tired. A hipster with a wiry dog on a leash comes out a side door, and I reach for the handle before it closes. Down a long hall I find a guard stand being presided over by a large woman with a pleasant but tired manner.

I tell her who I'm looking for.

"Oh?" She seems surprised. "He expecting you?"

"Nope." I smile.

She sticks out her lower lip, nods slowly, and reaches for the phone. Every movement appears to tax her.

"How's your day going?" I ask as she dials.

"It's going," she says, but she's clearly more interested in how this call might play out than in any chitchat with me. We wait a long time while the phone rings. "He's in there," she tells me.

"Hello?" I hear Seve's voice loud through the receiver at her ear.

"Hi. I've got—" The guard looks up at me.

I give her my name.

"Andrew, down here to see you."

There's a long pause on the line.

"Hello?" the guard says into the receiver.

"Down there?" comes the now halting voice on the other end of the phone. "With you?"

"Yes, sir," the guard says. "Want me to send him up?"

There's another pause, then, "Uh, okay. Send him up, please."

The guard disconnects the call and swings around in her chair. "He's got a few packages. Maybe you can bring them up."

"Sure." I follow her into the windowless room behind the podium, where she hands me one box and then another and another and another. My arms overflowing now, the guard holds the door for me.

"You can get the rest later," she says.

On the sixth floor I turn down a long hall with a vaguely nautical theme and pass one identical blue door after another. I drop a box and, bending to retrieve it, drop another, and then they all go tumbling like in a bad silent movie. Finally, at what I hope is the right apartment, I knock with my elbow.

The door opens a few inches. My friend stands there, incredulous, and cornered. "Dude?" Seve says. The one word contains a mix of dread, suspicion, affection, defensiveness, and warning. He is saying, in essence, "What the fuck are you trying to pull?"

"Man, if you came home drunk in this hallway, you'd never find the right apartment."

"What are you doing here?"

"I came to see you." I'm all smiles.

"I can see that." He's bent forward from the waist, leaning hard on the door handle, blocking the entrance. He has several days' growth of beard, is wearing blue warm-ups. His feet are bare.

"I'm coming in, so you might as well just open the door." I'm still smiling. "And take these fucking packages."

Seve shakes his head and backs away, a bewildered, embarrassed look on his face, his eyes lowered. The door swings open, and in an instant, I understand why Seve didn't want to let me in—and how Jeff Bezos became a billionaire. There are delivery boxes of all shapes and sizes. Everywhere. Piled high, tipped over, torn open, torn half open, empty, still sealed. And there are papers. Documents scattered and stacked high and precariously. And there are clothes, folded, thrown, some still in plastic bags. There is a narrow lane for limited movement through the space, but otherwise nothing of the floor is visible. Every surface is covered. The couch, save for one corner stacked strategically with pillows, is under a siege of clutter. I step in as best I can.

"Whoa, dude, you got a lot going on here. Where do you want these?" I say, referring to the boxes in my arms.

"Anywhere."

I let them drop. They would hit the floor, but there's so much already there that they just add to the pile.

Taller and bigger than me, Seve is cantilevered forward from the hip in a way I've never seen. "How's that back?" I ask, stepping forward to hug my friend.

"What are you doing here?" he says again, shaking his head.

"I came to see you, to watch the game." Seve is a Baltimore Orioles fan, and his team is finally making a run at the playoffs after years of futility.

"They're not playing today."

"Yeah, I heard that on the radio when I was halfway here."

Seve tries to laugh, but it gets caught in his throat. Upon entering, I immediately told myself not to try to straighten anything, not to humiliate my friend. But in my nervous energy, excited to reconnect and shocked to witness the state of his apartment, I start to pick up and discard things. Anything.

After only a few minutes we both begin to settle, but a lot of life has happened since our last get-together. And it's plain to see that a lot of that life has not been kind to my friend.

Over the next few hours, I empty and break down thirty-six cardboard boxes and fill eleven large green trash bags while Seve sits on the lone cleared spot on the couch, extra pillows supporting his back, hardly able to turn or move.

"No, don't throw that out!" is his frequent lament.

"Seve, what the fuck even is this?" is mine.

In the boxes I find solar-powered phone chargers, car waste baskets, protein powders, outlet adapters, paper towels, clothes, gummies of all sorts, three different clock radios, water, COVID tests, vitamins and more vitamins, coat hangers, cleaning supplies, more clothes, solvents, nuts and seeds, smoke alarms, gloves and hats, a collapsible walking stick. It's easy to imagine Seve scrolling his sleepless nights away, clicking, "Buy now," in an effort to fill his frustrating and nearly paralyzed present while imagining a future of movement and possibility. Each purchase is an act of optimism, or at least a desperate hope.

We continue to chat all the while as I work, but I'm too excited, too busy masking my distress for my friend, and for how long he has evidently been suffering in this fashion, to really concentrate on what I'm saying. We call our mutual friend Eddie, and the three of us shout back and forth on the phone for a few minutes while I break down boxes. Eddie suggests Seve and I pick some dates and road trip down to him. We all agree, but I know something now that Eddie doesn't—a road trip, much less any other kind of excursion, is not on the immediate horizon for our friend Seve. And while Eddie has stayed in closer contact to

Seve than I have, talking sports and life, Eddie lives in Dallas. He hasn't seen our friend in years either.

As the light outside begins to fade, Seve says, "I can get Grubhub to deliver."

"I'm not eating that shit," I say, tossing out whatever my hands land on. When I've begun to tire, with only a fraction of visible improvement to show for my efforts, Seve relents and agrees to go out to dinner.

He moves quickly down the hall, leaning forward at a precarious angle. Only now do I silently wonder if even this might be too much for my once vital, powerful friend.

"Slow down, Seve," I say. "Do you have a cane or a walker or something?"

"I don't need that," he says and keeps moving. He sits while we wait the thirty seconds for the elevator.

There's a small Asian fusion restaurant around the side of his building. Seve lowers himself into a booth, and I slip in on the other side. Only one other table in the place is occupied. The food is lousy, and it doesn't matter. In this neutral spot, away from the evidence of the strain of his life, away from his prison, my friend relaxes. His spirits rise. In sensing this, so do mine.

For the next half hour we fall into a familiar routine. I begin to rail about my life—the humiliations of my work, the intensity of my marriage, the demands of my kids. I don't really mean any of it too seriously, and while there may be truth in my words, it's not *the* truth—only a facet of what's going on, and one skewed from my obviously warped perspective.

But here with my friend, I'm not constrained by fairness or the need for any kind of mature perspective. A thoughtful, considered, and balanced assessment is not needed. It's not even the point. I just need to vent and purge, and Seve traditionally gives me a long lead.

There's no one else to whom I might say such things and feel in no way self-conscious or the need to qualify my litany of complaints—he knows that I am committed to my work, that I adore my wife, that I'm a pushover for my children. But I'm letting rip, and it feels good—it feels like our friendship.

That I didn't know this tirade was coming or that I needed to let my spleen go to such a degree is the obvious result of me for too long stifling my yearning for such connection. As I talk, I can feel I'm coming home to myself.

Seve is more than relieved to not think of his condition and does what he always does when I go off like this—he laughs in my face.

"No, please," he says at one point, laughing hard. "Stop. You're hurting my back."

Night has long fallen by the time we're back in Seve's condo. Only one lamp seems to light. I unpacked light bulbs earlier—I locate them and swap out a few.

"I'm sorry you can't stay here…" Seve starts.

"Don't even finish that sentence, Severino," I tell him. "It's all good." I had thought I'd stay the night in Baltimore, at a nearby hotel, but I'm feeling more energized than I normally do at this hour. "I think I'm gonna head home tonight."

"You sure? It's late. Let me get you a hotel with my Marriott points."

But I fill and take out a few more garbage bags. At the door, I hug my friend.

"Thanks for coming down," Seve says. He means it.

"Thanks for letting me in," I say, matching his sincerity.

Merging onto I-95, I'm feeling not so much buoyant as I am solid in myself, present—my usual dislike of highway driving has been replaced by a sense of rhythm with the road. After a half hour, Seve calls to thank me again. An hour later he calls to thank me one more time. In another hour, a midnight moon rises golden and nearly round over the refineries, keeping me company as I roll up the ugliest road in America.

Baltimore, Maryland
Part 2

A study by the University of Kansas concluded that it takes two hundred hours to make a good friend.[1] Seve and I are well past that number, but it is also well documented that one of the most vital ingredients in close friendship is consistency. Showing up. While daily or even frequent face-to-face interaction may not be practical with someone who lives a few states away, it feels important to reestablish a more solid base of contact with Seve.

So a week after my first visit I'm fighting my way down the New Jersey Turnpike again. Once more, I'm arriving unannounced, since Seve canceled on me coming again so soon. After eighty miles on "the Black Dragon," I veer off for a quick detour in Philadelphia, to drop something off for my wife. Stopping at the Bluestone Lane coffee shop on Walnut Street in the shadow of Rittenhouse Square for a cup of hot water to drop my tea bag into, I stumble into a surprising conversation with an open-faced man wearing round glasses that frame a steady gaze. His name is Jules.

I mention I'm headed down to see an old friend, and why.

"That's good," Jules says decisively. "Friendship can be elusive. And there's a need to feel less alone." He sips his coffee and looks off for a long moment before adding, "We've a lot to learn as men."

Raised by his mother, Jules grew up with four sisters. "I played hockey as a kid and never got close to any of the guys on the team. I could have used some male mentors. I was more at home with female friends, more at ease in conversation with women. Still am. I've always felt like I'm peeking over the fence in my friendships with men. Like I was on the outside looking in. Maybe because my relationship with my father was distant, but it never felt like a natural fit." He considers for a moment. "I understand the context of male friendship more since the military."

Before retiring in 2015 to begin life as a professor at the Wharton School, Jules served twenty-two years on the US Air Force Special Warfare Pararescue Team—meaning besides being an elite battlefield soldier, he was a parachutist, scuba diver, rock climber, and licensed paramedic trained "to provide acute care in humanitarian situations as well as direct action in contested spaces." Besides extensive experience in obvious hot spots like Afghanistan and Iraq, his team was among the first "on the pile" at the World Trade Center on 9/11.

Jules's forthcoming manner and emotional generosity with a stranger are disarming. I mention Matthew and Eddie, John and Don, how I'd hoped to reconnect with them as well. And the disappointment I've felt in that failing to happen.

Jules nods. "I feel guilty how little time I've invested in my friends. It's not enough." Then he shrugs. "I recharge by being by myself."

"I can relate to that," I say. I also know it is not a trait that's particularly conducive to the nurturing and maintaining of friendships.

Back on the road and crossing into Maryland, I instruct Siri to call Seve. My number isn't blocked, yet Seve never answers when I call. Invariably he calls back in a few minutes.

"I'm coming in!" I shout by way of greeting.

"When, today?" Seve asks, poorly veiled panic in his voice.

"Yeah, baby. Brace yourself."

"Where are you?"

"Maryland somewhere. Half hour out."

"Jesus." Seve tries to chuckle.

"See you then!" I shout and hang up before there can be any more discussion on the matter.

I fill nine trash bags and empty and break down twenty-seven boxes. Opening one of the new spray disinfectants, I'm defeated trying to clean the kitchen. I attempt to organize the scores of prescription bottles on the counter. I come across a bottle of veterinary pills and a written prescription for someone named Calbert.

"When did your dog die?" I ask.

"About five years ago."

I hold up the prescription. "What the fuck, Seve?"

"No judgment, dude, no judgment."

He's right. Seve knows the situation he's in. There's no need for me to shame and humiliate him. I pivot back to humor and do my best to ignore the pink elephant buried under all this clutter.

It's easier to get him out of the house this time.

"I'm not going back to that shithole," I say after Seve suggests the same Asian fusion restaurant we went to a week earlier. We get in my car and drive a few parking lots over to the Bayside Cantina, a Mexican restaurant. It's just as lifeless as the last place, the food just as bad. Once again, it doesn't matter.

Seve has always relished revisiting past escapades—"Hey, do you remember..." starts many of his sentences, and always has. Unlike many people who relive the past from a place of wistful yearning or melancholy, I always know Seve is relaxed and happy whenever he recalls the glory days. Only now, with so few current adventures and the prospect of future ones in question, the phrase takes on a different tone—at least for me.

We talk again about the day I met my wife in the west of Ireland, to which Seve was the only witness.

"Talk about a third wheel." He laughs.

"You didn't even try to stop me," I scold him.

"One look and that was over, my friend," he says, summing up my instantaneous connection with Dolores. "You've had that experience. Not many people do." Dolores and my union is something my friend has always validated and admired.

As we finish our bad tacos, talk shifts to Seve's medical condition and what he calls his "game plan," but there's an undercurrent tonight.

"I used to think I adapted well to change…" Seve says, but the thought goes unfinished.

I watch my friend. I've known him long enough to know what he's doing in the silence—pivoting away from the slippery slope of despair and rallying himself the way a high school coach might give his team a pep talk. Finally, he speaks. "I'm gonna get rid of all the shit. Keep one suit, one tie. Get a good routine and not succumb."

The bill is placed on the table.

"My dad's gonna pay," I tell the waitress, and push the check toward Seve.

Seve laughs and shakes his head. "Still works," he says, referring to a well-worn line of ours.

I hand over my credit card while Seve's use of the word "succumb" rings in my head. I'm distressed for my friend. Seve has always been one of the most gregarious people I know. An ever-charming extrovert, his enforced isolation is heavy emotional weight for him to carry. He has a mountain to climb and no partner, no kids—he will need his friends. The three a.m. thoughts must be terrifying. No wonder he spends the small hours ordering online, distracting himself.

Back at his place I'm touched and surprised when Seve invites me to sleep on his couch. "You just got it clean," he explains. But I'm finding it difficult tonight to remain relentlessly upbeat.

I regret leaving, but I have little left to offer at the moment.

At the door, after I embrace my friend, he laughs. "Hey, do you remember how happy you were dancing that jig at your wedding?"

I sleep poorly at a local hotel and in the morning fight my own sense of deterioration by doing exercises I often neglect. In the middle of a set of push-ups, I suddenly begin to sob. The word "succumb" circles back again. Then Dylan Thomas's line to "rage, rage against the dying of the light" pops into my head. I call Seve but know he's finally asleep, having no doubt been up most of the night pacifying himself, clicking "Buy now."

While I'm driving north on I-95, construction on the Delaware Memorial Bridge has closed two lanes and is causing trucks doing eighty miles per hour to push over the dotted white lines and into my lane. While stressful, I don't indulge in the kind of anxiety that I might typically allow under these conditions. My mood is sober, with no need for self-dramatizing emotional theatrics. This morning I'm acutely aware of the impermanence we all face.

It's two weeks later and I've just gotten off the train. It's five p.m. I call Seve. There's no answer, of course, but no call back either.

At five thirty I arrive at his building and call him again. Still no response. The idea of battling down I-95 one more time filled me with dread, so I let Amtrak get me here. Again, I'm arriving unannounced. Despite Seve assuring me how much my visits mean to him, he's canceled on me twice since my last visit. I enter the building and approach the guard stand. The same heavyset woman greets me. She's still pleasant, still exhausted.

"You can just go on up," she says.

Grabbing an armload of boxes from the storage room, I'm in the elevator and then I'm walking down that long, blue-doored, vaguely nautical-themed hallway. I knock. There's no answer. I pound on the door and call my friend's name. Still no reply. I return to the guard stand.

"He hasn't gone out, has he?"

She screws her face up, as if to say, "Are you fucking crazy?"

"You seen him lately?"

"He came down yesterday, to get some boxes."

I go back up and pound on the door again, calling loud. I'm surprised none of the neighbors come out to see what all the fuss is about. I press my ear to the door; no sound comes from the apartment. I slump down and sit against the wall opposite his door. In time I call our friend Eddie.

"Oh, shit," he says. "How long have you been there?"

"About an hour."

We discuss calling the police.

I suggest we hold off and then go to get some dinner a few blocks away. After, sitting on a bench eating gelato, I try to reconcile eating ice cream while my friend could be locked in his room, in trouble, or worse.

I return to his building and look up from outside. His windows are dark, the curtains drawn. I go up and pound on the door again, shouting, "SEVE! SEVE!" By now it's ten p.m., five hours since I arrived.

I go down one more time and speak to the manager of the building, who readily agrees to come up with me and open the apartment. She places the key in the lock, swings the door open, and steps back for me to enter. The air is stale, but the air is always stale. The room is dark, and I snap on the lights. Calling out, "SEVE! SEVE!" I creep around the corner, aware of the possibility that I might see something I will never be able to forget. What I cleaned two weeks earlier has been returned to its previous state, but I'm not concerned with clutter. I approach his bedroom and, using the flashlight on my phone, see Seve sprawled across the bed, on his back, his mouth agape. Then his chest rises and falls.

"It's okay," I call out to the manager, who has remained by the door.

She leaves, and I attempt to rouse my friend. Seve tries to fight his way back through whatever fog is enveloping him. He manages a few words but nothing coherent, then falls back to sleep. I stand over him and watch. His breathing is deep and regular. I call Eddie.

"Thank Christ," he says.

I stay around for a bit to be sure Seve's breathing remains strong and try to clean up a little, but my heart isn't in it. I feel foolish for being so concerned, for overreacting, but I'm also mad at Seve. How the fuck did things get so bad? Eventually, I crack open a door to his balcony to allow in some air, and leave.

Returning to the same hotel I stayed at before, I sleep poorly again. In the morning I'm up early and walking along the waterfront, trying to clear my head.

In a cramped marina, a lone man is working on a small sailboat with the word *Friendship* stenciled on the back—its mast is broken. I brush the cheap metaphor away. Trying to offer some encouragement, I call out, "Nice boat."

The man barely raises his head and grunts a response.

He's right. Who am I to bestow blessings? What am I trying to prove? And to whom? What am I really doing coming down here to Baltimore? Trying to make up for time lost? Or trying to play big shot? Savior? If Seve doesn't want me to come down—and he doesn't seem to, since he's canceled on me every time—then don't come down.

I walk on. There is no sun. The air is raw. That I often prefer my own company to being with others has certainly played a large part in how I came to be in the position of having not seen my friends in so long, but I can't remember the last time I felt this way. I very rarely feel lonely, but this feels a lot like loneliness.

A small dog at the end of a long leash races toward me. I bend to pet her, and she gets tangled around my ankles. The frustrated owner tries to smile as we unwrap, and they move on.

Maybe I'm too late. Perhaps too much time and life have gone over the dam. Others have lives that they're living—they aren't waiting for me to show up. Who am I to announce on a whim after so many years that I suddenly want to nurture what should have been tended to long ago?

But staring across the harbor to Baltimore's iconic Domino Sugar sign, it feels now or never. I reach for my phone and call Matthew. It rings a long time. I'm suddenly very hungry.

"Sport!" Matthew's voice shouts over the line.

I have no idea where that nickname came from, but Matthew and I have called each other Sport for more than thirty years. The warmth of his greeting settles me.

"I know you're swamped," I begin, my tone somber, then ask my friend if I can come take him to dinner.

Maybe he can hear something in my voice, but after the briefest hesitation Matthew says simply, "Love to, Sport. I got a game tonight and shit tomorrow. Just give me a couple of days."

I could take the train home and then fly down, but I'm already in motion, already halfway to Lexington, Kentucky. And if I do return home, I'm worried I won't get right back out—afraid I'll fall under the demands and stresses of my day-to-day.

"The way I drive, it'll take me a few days anyway," I say.

"You're driving?"

"Well, I'm already in Baltimore."

Matthew pauses. "Cool. But you're gonna have to drive through West Virginia and eastern Kentucky," he says with a trace of horror in his voice. A self-professed "Jew from Long Island," Matthew has never fully embraced his current surroundings.

"I've never been there. It'll be interesting to see."

He laughs, then signs off. "Good luck, Sport."

Before I can think myself out of it, I rent a car, and within an hour I'm heading west.

Matthew

Harpers Ferry, West Virginia

Many people find getting behind the wheel relaxing. The thrill of the open road. Radio up loud. Windows down with the wind in your hair and troubles at your back. The notion that we can just drive away from our cares and woes is a seductive one—the belief that there's no problem so great that it can't be solved by a pocket full of cash and a tank full of gas. And the feeling of chasing the sun across the country calls to mind a distinctly American sense of freedom. Head west young man, the saying goes. (Does this apply to the not so young as well?)

Unfortunately, I am not one of those road-trip-loving people. There's the stiffness in my lower back from sitting behind the wheel for so long, and the tightness in my hip. And of course there's the monotony of the road. The questionable cleanliness of motel beds. The bad food. But it's the persistent sense of peril I experience on a highway with eighteen-wheelers surging past that creates a near-constant simmer of anxiety that I dread most. With age comes increased awareness of the unpredictability and precarious nature of life. I've known and heard of too many people who died behind the wheel—victims of a freak accident, of being in the exact wrong place at the exact wrong time. And since I recently indulged in looking at a single roadside pileup online, my Instagram feed has become clogged with reels of errant tires flying into windshields, trucks overturning across four lanes, cars flipping like playthings. Add to this that I know nothing about how the vehicle I'm driving works, and if I were to break down, especially on some remote section of road far out in the hinterland, I would be stranded, helpless.

Regardless, I'm on the road. And with time on my hands, coupled with my disdain of interstate highways, it's an easy decision to avoid I-70 and slip back onto Route 40. I pass row houses with dented aluminum awnings. Rusting and mismatched furniture clutter brick porches. An entire block has been boarded up. West Baltimore has long been one of the country's most disenfranchised neighborhoods. At a red light a cold wind blows in through my open window, and I stare at a hand-painted sign in front of a clapboard house offering fried chicken for sale. An overturned tricycle sits in the driveway behind a deeply dented Honda. A work-program cleanup team, a ragtag cluster of men in yellow vests holding dark plastic bags, pluck trash from the center divider, while on the car radio a panel discusses the idea of reparations and the failure of reconstruction after the Civil War.

Route 40 forces me briefly onto I-70, and Seve calls.

"I have this crazy memory, or maybe it was a dream. Were you here shining a flashlight?"

"Yup."

"Then when I saw the door to the balcony was open a bit, I was like…"

I explain the evening, my arrival, my pounding on the door. "I was scared, Seve."

He explains how he hadn't slept at all the previous two nights and had finally taken a sleeping pill.

"Well, Jesus, dude, you were fucking out."

We laugh.

"I'm turning around here," I say. "I'll head back now."

"No, no," Seve demurs. "I need to get some more sleep. Go see Matthew. But, Andrew"—Seve rarely uses my name, and he does so now with feeling—"thanks for checking."

Relieved, I carry on.

A little over an hour west of Baltimore sits Harpers Ferry, just across the Potomac in West Virginia. From my schoolboy history I have a vague recollection that Harpers Ferry was the site of abolitionist John Brown's ill-fated raid on the armory, which helped to bring the issue of slavery to the heart of the national debate. And so as I drift out into America with a few days to kill before meeting up with Matthew, this thin strand of schoolboy history is enough to keep me tethered—I head that way.

US Route 340 has become rural and crosses the Appalachian Trail. At the Potomac I can see my destination just a mile upriver. But a twenty-five-mile, forty-five-minute detour takes me deep into Virginia instead—over rolling farmland and fallow fields and fenced-in meadows with horses grazing. A forty-foot billboard in the cutout of a rifle announces a shooting range. When I pass a Waffle House, I know I'm in the South.

This part of the country has never been clear in my mind. Virginia, West Virginia, Ohio, Pennsylvania, and Maryland all feel crammed up into one another. West Virginia sits largely to the *north* of Virginia, while a strand of it crawls up the west side of Pennsylvania. Coastal Maryland seems barely on solid ground at all, yet manages to slither around the top of West Virginia. And someone decided that Pennsylvania is in the east, while next door Ohio is the heart of the Midwest. West Virginia and Virginia are southern, even as longitudinally parallel Maryland is mid-Atlantic. And they all seem within a four iron of one another.

I take a rise and see a lone figure wearing a hard hat standing in the middle of the road, a stop sign on a stick in hand. A single orange traffic cone sits at his feet. I see no other roadworks crew. No people at all. I approach and ease to a stop beside the young man wearing the hard hat. He's in his early twenties, chubby, has carrot-colored hair and an unkempt, patchy beard that frizzes out like wire. I lower the window. His name is Cory and he's from nearby Hillsboro, a few miles south. Cory has a two-year-old daughter named Mary Grace, who lives even closer.

"But I only get to see her when they let me," he explains.

The wind blows through the trees.

I wonder how far ahead the unseen roadwork is.

"They're down there a ways," Cory says.

We sit.

"I'm headed to Harpers Ferry. Nice town?"

"Never been."

"It's pretty close, though, right?"

Cory nods. "I think they got good places to shop."

We're silent again.

I wonder if Cory's ever traveled out of state.

He shakes his head, "I never do much 'cept work and go to the Walmart." His tone is resigned, fatalistic. He seems only distantly interested in his own experience.

"Just hang out with your friends, huh?" I ask, trying to encourage him.

He shrugs. "I don't git out too much. I stick to myself."

We sit with that too.

Finally, Cory's walkie-talkie squawks, and he spins the stop sign to "Slow." "You can go," he tells me. I want to say something to Cory, something to buoy his spirits or light a fire under him, but I'm not sure what. Driving off, I watch Cory grow smaller and smaller in the rearview mirror while he stares off motionless.

I finally slide into what feels like the back door to Harpers Ferry, sitting on the point where the Potomac and the Shenandoah Rivers meet. Like many Civil War or Revolutionary era towns, Harpers Ferry feels not so much a living place but a site of amusement in ye olde guise whose main purpose is mining an idea of the past for profit today. After a cursory walk-through of the John Brown Museum, I'm looking for food.

Picking a restaurant at random on High Street, I settle in at the bar for an overpriced burger. The walls around me are covered with mounted muskets and fading maps, flags and paintings of Civil War generals. I fall into conversation with a young man who works here but has just come in to collect his pay.

His name is Joseph. He's twenty-three, black hair, full eyebrows, olive skin; he's a local boy who went away to school and has come home.

"I don't think any of my friends are from college. All are from growing up."

"You see them often?" I ask just to hit the ball back across the net.

"Pretty much every day. Or every few days."

"So, often enough."

He nods. "I'm not married or anything yet, so I still have a lot of people I haven't lost touch with. I live alone, and the demons start to take over. It can start to feel like solitary confinement, especially with the internet. So I need to do something."

"Ah, the internet."

"Yeah, it gets lonely for sure. Social interaction scratches an itch, like working out does. If I don't do it, I feel worse. It's definitely something I need every day, or I go crazy."

"That's a pretty insightful thing to realize about yourself," I say, dipping a French fry in some ketchup.

"I've thought about it a lot. What does a person need? Every day."

"And?"

"You need to eat well, exercise, have a hobby or passion, and connection. You can take away any one and you suffer, but take away social interaction and you fall apart the fastest. That's the person that would kill themselves first."

"What do you do with your friends around here?"

"Well, with guys it's a more lighthearted thing. We play video games, go to the gym. I'm in an indie rock band, so we play music."

"And that's different from what you'd do with women?"

"Sure, with guys we just distract each other. I wouldn't say to them that I'm lonely, for example, or sad. Where I would with a girl. Or with a guy, if I did say I was depressed, I'd have to do it in a laughing way. I might say the words but never show the emotion. Where with girls I'd let them know what I was feeling."

His phone rings. Joseph silences it without looking at who's calling.

"Feel free to grab that," I say.

"No, I'm enjoying this. It's interesting."

I'm impressed not only by Joseph's self-possession, but by his easy candor. So I press on. "Do you ever wish you could express your feelings in a vulnerable way to a guy?"

"No. Maybe if I could reset all of society, I'd be more comfortable. If everything were equal, maybe. But I don't know that

I'd want to be in that dynamic. If I consoled a guy who opened up, I'd be uncomfortable. Being vulnerable in front of a guy just feels wrong."

"You're really direct and open with me right now," I say.

"We're talking about it analytically," he says. "I've thought about this. Maybe it's just me or maybe it's societal. Say a guy tells me his grandmother died. I wouldn't know what to say. I don't know how to console him."

"And with a woman you would?"

"Yeah."

"Do you think there's some kind of anxiety about a sexual component in that vulnerability?"

Joseph considers. "Maybe there's a homo...homophobic quality. But I don't know."

"Guys seem to get stuck right there a lot," I say.

"Well, with my dad, when his parents died, I had no idea how to comfort him. I don't think I did at all. But when my mom's mother died, I gave her a hug. I could comfort her."

Joseph seems so clear-headed about the topic, so astute. Certainly, far more than I was at his age.

"I think it's also cultural," Joseph goes on. "I'm half Filipino, half white. The white side of my family is very individualistic, less family-focused. On my Filipino side, my mother sees her sisters almost every day, the cousins are always over, my grandmother lived with us for seven years till she died. I think there's a whole cultural component to how social we are, and it affects our health. My grandparents on the white side got Alzheimer's. Neither on the Filipino side did."

My phone rings. Joseph nods toward it. "I gotta go get my money anyway," he says and heads into the back office.

It's Eddie.

"You talk to Seve?"

"Yeah, he called this morning. We had a laugh."

"Well, not anymore."

Apparently, the longer Seve sat with my intrusion, the more upset he became. How dare I barge in? At the front desk they should never have allowed it. Only his sister has the right to enter his apartment.

"Oh, shit." I understand Seve's reaction. If the situation were reversed, I would feel ashamed, humiliated.

"Yeah."

I call Seve. Naturally, he doesn't answer. I leave a message saying I've spoken to Eddie, I want to apologize, please call. He doesn't.

Agitated and anxious now, I need to move. I pay and get up to go. Joseph comes back from the kitchen. "Enjoy West Virginia," he says. "It's a real undiscovered gem."

I assure Joseph I will, but now my mind is elsewhere.

"And I was just making a tiered list of my friends on my phone," he says. "I'm not done yet, but it's really interesting. A lot of friends come and go like the seasons."

Taking up Route 340 south, I pass vineyards with dead leaves hanging from lifeless vines. Tilting headstones cling to a sloping hill beyond a wrought iron fence. The carcass of a large deer has been pulled to the side of the winding, two-lane road. I cross Turkey Run Creek. Cattle pick at patchy grass in a rock-littered field. Far to the north, wind turbines line a ridge, lifeless.

Heading west over a rise on the rural two-lane John Marshall Highway, I pull into the New Star Market—Gas, Outfitter, and BBQ all in one—hoping to revive my spirits with a cup of tea. A tiny, elderly man is restocking the white bread. He calls himself Mr. Park. In a very strong accent, he lets me know he came from South Korea in 1985.

"I went back for Olympics in '88, but never again. I don't know anything about Korea, except what I see on Korean soap opera."

I ask for a cup of hot water. Then hold a tea bag aloft to Mr. Park, indicating the reason for my request.

"Tea," he says, then nods. "Good."

Mr. Park sets a large steaming Styrofoam container onto the counter. "You pay me twenty-five cent."

He's worked in this seemingly random corner of the world, so far from home, for twenty years. "My friend owns it," he tells me by way of explanation. Then, while elaborating on his own situation, Mr. Park unwittingly speaks to the truth I've been trying to deny for too long and why I'm out here on the road at all—"Need to have friends. Life is too hard without friends."

Elkins, West Virginia

West Virginia is the only state to lie completely within the Appalachian Mountain range. Winding, rising, falling, sweeping—the roads are never flat or straight. And nearly all of them feel deserted. Twisting south on Route 32, the dying autumnal light in the Monongahela National Forest is gauzy. The western horizon is aqua, then pink, then violet. These mountains, while not approaching the grandeur of the Rockies, offer an experience that's both immediate and vast, simultaneously claustrophobic and expansive, peak after peak after peak receding. The constant rise and fall of the road continually alters perspective, and the ever-changing vista feels like a distinct and singular American pleasure.

In the gloaming, a dozen deer gingerly make their way from the woods. I slow and then stop to let them cross the road. A silver sliver of a moon is rising.

Seve didn't call back all day. Normally I wouldn't think twice about that, but my entering his apartment yesterday felt anything but normal. I think of my other neglected, atrophying friendships—about what I'm doing out here on the road in the gathering Appalachia darkness.

I flash on the muted ache I felt coming from Cory during our brief roadside encounter when he said, "I don't git out too much. I stick to myself." The words of Joseph at the restaurant in Harpers Ferry come back—"It gets lonely for sure." And the remarks by Jules, the air force pararescue officer I met back in Philadelphia—"Friendship can be elusive. There's a need to feel less alone. We've a lot to learn as men."

What's going on?

The deer have picked their way into the trees, been absorbed into the blackness. I need to find a place for the night. Instead I ease my car off the side of the road. I reach for my phone and start scrolling, looking for answers.

Men, it turns out, have lost the knack for friendship.

Fifteen percent of men confess to having no close friends at all, up from three percent in 1990,[1] while less than half of all men say they are satisfied with how many friends they have.[2] Only one in five men report receiving any form of emotional support from a friend in the prior week,[3] and among those with only a high school diploma, twenty-four percent of men admit to having no friends whatsoever.[4] The situation is particularly dire for the young. One study found that seventy-nine percent of Gen Zers and seventy-one percent of millennials confess to being lonely.[5]

Meanwhile, Joseph may have been right in suspecting that his grandparents' mental states were related to how social they were. There's a staggering fifty percent elevated risk in developing Alzheimer's,[6] a twenty-nine percent increased chance of heart disease, and a thirty-two percent increased instance of stroke for those with "poor social relationships."[7] I'm clicking fast now, the statistics piling up. Social isolation exceeds the health risks of obesity, inactivity, air pollution, consuming more than six alcoholic drinks per day, and smoking more than fifteen cigarettes a day.[8] And men are four times more likely to take their own lives than women.[9] The surgeon general has declared an epidemic of loneliness.[10]

"What the fuck," I say to the empty car.

By the time I put down my phone, the young moon has climbed the black sky. A gaudy display of stars blink beyond the high bare branches of dormant trees. Confirmed in the need to reconnect with my friends, I shift into drive and ease my way deeper into Appalachia.

I settle in Elkins, with a population of about seven thousand—enough to create a sense of community, yet distinctly small enough for people to have made a clear choice in how they want to live.

In Beanders Bar, I stumble upon that staple of off-night promotion, the trivia contest. I fall into conversation with the bartender, Rodney, a local boy and a bridge inspector by day. Beside me at the bar, Chris and Renee struggle for an answer in tonight's quiz and solicit my help. I know less than they do. Chris and Renee moved down from Michigan for his work in the Park Service. Affable in a Midwestern way, they're welcoming to a stranger, yet guarded—interlopers themselves in this community.

"How long you been here?" I ask.

"A year," Renee says.

"Made any friends?"

Chris looks around. "Well, no enemies, anyway. Families go back five, six generations. We're outsiders. But people are nice enough."

I supply my lone correct trivia answer of the evening, sit back with disproportionate satisfaction, and Rodney leans over the bar to offer me a high five.

"Ah," Renee says wryly, "the lowest common denominator of male intimacy."

Only later do I wonder—and wish I had asked—what a woman in a similar situation might have done instead to demonstrate camaraderie, solidarity, affection, even intimacy—because obviously, men and women tend to handle and treat their friendships differently.

I recall my wife once commenting on one of my friends, how he seemed a bit "slippery."

"I'm sure you're right." I shrugged.

"And...?"

"He's my friend," I said. It was the end of the discussion.

Nietzsche, not famous for being the most gregarious of German philosophers, summed it up nicely: "Love is blind, friendship closes its eyes."

Yet if that had been a friend of Dolores's, there is every chance that she and the friend would have felt the need to talk out this perceived character flaw, its effects and repercussions. It might have required a cup of tea, a difficult conversation, possibly a good cry, followed by hugs and a recommitment and pledge to deeper friendship. This observation may seem clichéd or read like an unfair stereotype, even sexist, but I've seen exactly this in action, and I admire the emotional rigor of both parties—envy it, even. But the experience in most of my male friendships is that, unless the transgression is so great or character flaw too extreme, we generally incorporate them into the dynamic of the friendship, usually without even an acknowledgment, and move on.

Though there are occasional instances where the perceived flaw rises to such a level that the friendship cannot withstand it.

I had one such friend. I'll call him Simon. Our friendship began on a movie set. And work remained a peripheral part of our interactions for several years as we grew closer. I sought Simon out whenever I was in London. Occasionally, I stayed at his place. He did the same when he came to New York. We spoke often on the phone. At one point Simon partnered up with someone and began to produce movies. I had gotten into directing. He asked me to read a film script. I responded to it positively and flew to London to meet. There were a few discussions. Then things went quiet, and soon there was vague talk of someone else possibly directing the project. "What's up?" I asked.

I couldn't really object to Simon and his partner going with someone else. I knew the caprices and disappointments of show business far too well to take them personally. It required a simple, and awkward, conversation. The friendship might have endured a period of distance, but we would have survived. Instead, Simon skirted the question and asked me to read another script they had on a shelf and were "excited" about. I knew this was merely intended to pacify me and divert my attention as the first project went away.

But we were friends, good friends. What was happening? Was our friendship not worth the truth? Or at least a better lie?

"Oh. Um, send the script" was all I could muster on the phone and hung up.

Simon never called me again, nor I him.

Although this happened years ago, I still think of Simon. I'm sorry such a close friendship ended the way it did—it was a painful loss. Yet had Simon admitted he was aware this would hurt me, had I acknowledged how merciless I knew producers needed to be to get a movie made, had we behaved with even a portion of the sensitivity for each other's feelings that my wife and her female friends do, Simon and I might still be friends.

Or maybe I just had it wrong with Simon.

No less than Aristotle said that "differences between friends most frequently arise when the nature of the friendship is not what they think it is."[11] The Greek philosopher dissected the issue of friendship and asserted that there were three distinct types—utility-based friends, which might include work friends, who both understand and benefit from the exchange. Then there are pleasure-based friends, with whom we share a common and pleasing activity, be it dinner parties or baseball, or they might be people we simply enjoy being around—maybe they're funny. The third type of friendship, and what Aristotle called "perfect friends," are character-based friendships. These are the friends in whom we see their inherent good, and they see ours. These are friends who are aware of their feelings for each other and take pleasure in that awareness. These friendships make us better people. The first and second types of friendship can evolve into the third, but certainly not always. Perhaps the problem between Simon and me was as simple as I believed the friendship to be in one category, while he understood it to be in another.

Point Pleasant, West Virginia

The following morning I'm in Scottie's Diner over on Seventh Street. Formica tables, a few booths, cheap venetian blinds. A handwritten sign taped to the bulletin board announces that Scottie is looking for a cook. Someone must be in the kitchen since the place is humming at eight a.m. A middle-aged woman prowls the floor, refilling coffee, taking orders, dishing out remarks. Another is behind the register, making change and barking into the phone. "Sunday would be great, George. Appreciate it. And I'll get these coffees ready for you now." A third woman comes out of the kitchen to fetch a gallon of milk from the refrigerator in the corner and hurries back through the swinging door.

Eight middle-aged and older men, seven of them wearing mesh baseball caps, all of them still wearing their coats, occupy the large table in the center of the room. They sip coffee, talk. The man without a hat leaves with little fanfare, the way people do when they know they'll see one another tomorrow, and the day after, and the day after that. Within minutes, another man, bearing a striking resemblance to the scarecrow from *The Wizard of Oz*, enters and without ceremony fills the recently vacated seat.

I surprise myself by wanting to walk over and introduce myself, to join their group. It's not something I would ever consider under normal circumstances, but out here on the road, chasing what has begun to feel like the ghosts of friendship, trying to reclaim what I hope I haven't lost, I'm looking for something.

I've often sought and found answers to my questions on the road. Travel has, in many ways, been the university of my life. Looked at in this light, it's no wonder I became a travel writer. Travel has taught me about myself and my place in the world. About my relation to others. Experience tells me that the farther from home I go, the more at home in myself I tend to feel. On the road, habits are replaced by curiosity. Certainty yields to inquisition. And in this bustling room of strangers who live a life very different from mine, there are people who know things I don't, who might offer me insight, might help me uncover, or discover, some of what friendship has to offer and help me clarify what it means to me, what place it has in my life.

But Chris's words from the bar last night rattle in my head—I'm from away, an outsider.

I stay put, but then fall into conversation with the couple at the next table. Even sitting down, I can see that Kevin is very tall. He wears a full beard. Jennifer is blond, with glasses—she's well turned out.

"Quite a buzz in here," I say.

"There is." Kevin nods. "Every morning."

"Is that the brain trust?" I ask, indicating the large group of men in the center of the room.

"They'd like to think so," Jennifer says, rolling her eyes. Then she softens and clarifies what I might have learned had I summoned the courage to interject myself into their fold. "At least they've got each other."

And that seems to be the key. During last evening's roadside deep-dive, I came upon the results of a recent eighty-five-year study by Harvard University[1] that concluded the number one factor in a longer, healthier, happier life is not diet or exercise, or meaningful work, but a positive and consistent connection to community. It appears that the "brain trust" around the table already knew something it took the Ivy League nearly a century of study to realize.

I could drive due west and be at Matthew's for a late lunch. But since I have nearly two days before he's freed up, I turn south from Elkins on Route 250. I pass churches, revival houses, outreach ministries. I pass roadkill, gas stations, abandoned gas stations. Unincorporated communities appear and are just as quickly forgotten. A Dollar General store anchors any more substantial settlement. The winding road is picturesque, but I'm distracted, still bothered about Seve, that I humiliated him. Yet his isolation worries me. Still too early for him to be awake, I hope he'll call anyway.

I pass through tiny and impoverished Mingo. A scrappy dog chases me down the road for a long while, barking wildly. I make a sharp left onto Route 66.

Up and then down and around, on a narrow valley floor deep in the mountains and surrounded by steep and densely forested hills, I come upon the company town of Cass, a settlement of neatly arranged white buildings laid out above a railroad track in 1901 by the West Virginia Pulp and Paper Company. Timber from Cheat Mountain was processed here and taken away by train. What made this timber—even now barely accessible—so much more desirable than any of the identical-looking timber I've passed all morning escapes me. The mill closed in the sixties, and the state bought the site.

It's always disheartening when unique and once vital places, ripe for reinvention, are simply handed over to the tourist trade and repackaged for bite-size exploitation. Only there's no one here. The small parking lot is empty, the rows of white houses, silent. It is a town set waiting for the actors to arrive.

Inside the sprawling general store selling trinkets and cheap china, Muzak plays loud. A fair-haired young man in his early twenties with nose piercings and tattoos down his arm stands alone behind a cafeteria food station. An unidentifiable combination of smells waft out. I approach the young man, the only person in sight. His name tag says "Bud."

"What goes on here in Cass, Bud?" I ask stupidly.

In time, Bud, who is doing nothing, glances up at me across the trays of food. He appears neither surprised to see me nor the least bit interested.

"I don't know," he says slowly.

"Really?"

"When the railroad runs..." he begins, but the rest of Bud's thought seems to fail him. Then he concludes, "But it doesn't run now."

"You mean doesn't run this time of year or anymore?" I ask.

"Huh?"

"Is the train shut down for the season, or forever?"

"Yeah."

I try a different tack.

"Who comes here?"

"Nobody much."

Our conversation, such as it is, falters.

"Have a good day, Bud."

Pause.

"Okay."

Nearly defeated by this exchange, I retrace my steps out of the valley of the damned and take up Route 219, past fields with dry brown corn stalks, plowed-under fields, uncultivated fields. I see few other cars and continue south to Louisburg. I have no business here, nor anywhere else in West Virginia. Yesterday I was enlivened by a sense of discovery. Today I wonder what the hell I'm doing. Matthew sounded busy anyway. Maybe I should just go home.

I eat a solitary lunch, then loop north and west. The elevated road tracking the Kanawha River snakes through steep, pine-covered hills. Around the next bend, beyond the next hill, smoke fills the sky. The road climbs and sweeps and reveals a semi-trailer hastily pulled to the shoulder of the road. It's on fire. Ferocious flames from the engine lick high into the sky, feeding on themselves. The smoke caused by the inferno turns day to night in the confined valley. No police or rescue are on the scene. The driver of the truck is nowhere in sight.

Seve still hasn't called back by late in the day. I've crossed the state and find myself in a town called Point Pleasant, West Virginia. I know nothing about this place. The only reason I'm here is because there's a bridge over the river to Ohio. Tomorrow I'll slice across a corner of the Buckeye State and drop down into Kentucky, continuing south to Lexington and Matthew in time for dinner.

A slow drive up and down a deserted Main Street reveals once handsome buildings hinting at a more vital past. On the corner of Fourth and Main, I come upon the formerly regal Lowe Hotel. It looks abandoned, but the autumnal evening has come on quickly and I need a place to sleep. I try the door, and it swings open.

Built in 1901, the place, including its furnishings, appears not to have changed much since then. A lone middle-aged woman in a floral dress with blond hair from a bottle is sunk deep in a faded, lavender armchair in the corner of the lobby beside a green glass lamp. I nod in her direction, and her eyes follow me as I approach the front desk. No one is behind the counter. I gently tap the silver bell and wait.

Time passes.

"Can I help you?" the woman from the corner croaks, breaking the long silence.

I turn. "I'm looking for a room for the night."

"We're full."

"Really?"

"Sorry."

Baffled, I turn to go.

When I'm almost back through the door, the woman in the corner calls after me, "Where you from?"

"New York," I answer, my hand still on the knob.

"I can find you a room," she says, and hoists herself up.

"Great."

She crosses the threadbare rug and makes her way behind the counter. A wall full of keys dangle in cubbies behind her. "Thought you might be local and just looking for a place to spend the night."

Always pleased when I can pass for a local, I wonder why they might be undesirable.

"A lot of homeless here," she explains.

"I see." I promise myself I'll find a laundromat tomorrow.

Returning to the car to grab my bag, I glance across the street to a storefront museum dedicated to Point Pleasant's main attraction.

On November 15, 1966, four teenagers were out joyriding and came upon a large humanoid creature with glowing red eyes and a pair of wings. The two couples beat it back to town and told the local newspaper. Then when the town's Silver Bridge spanning the Ohio River collapsed soon after, killing forty-six people, suspicion was raised about a possible connection with the mysterious entity now being called...Mothman. Over the next few years others reported seeing the strange being. A book was written about the creature. Then someone in Hollywood thought this was a good idea for a movie starring Richard Gere. Legend grew, and at one point up to twenty-five thousand people descended on Point Pleasant for the annual Mothman festival.

"Mothman saved this town," says Brett, who works behind the counter at the two-room museum cluttered with newspaper articles, posters, and seemingly unrelated other spooky things. He has a round, pale face and greasy black hair with dark circles under his eyes. It doesn't look like Brett gets outside much. He appears to be in his late twenties. "I was here when most of Main Street was boarded up. This was a desolate spot."

I mention the lack of street life now.

"We're here, all right," he says. "But you know, we're not necessarily country folk, but we're county."

I'm not really sure what that means.

"Everybody knows everybody," Brett explains, "although most young people couldn't carry on a conversation."

"You must have friends, though."

"If you ask me friends, real friends, I'd say I got seven or eight friends I can call and depend on anytime."

I nod, impressed.

Brett thinks a moment. "Actually, there's only two I'd call in the middle of the night, if you know what I mean."

"Two middle-of-the-night calls ain't bad," I assure him.

Brett thinks some more. "I'd call them each for different things... Well... I'd definitely call one of them..."

Before Brett can equivocate himself out of any friends at all, I return to my hotel.

Up a flight of creaking, sloping stairs, past a grand piano in the parlor lounge, I find my room. The bed is worryingly concave. The drawstring on the curtain is broken. The window is painted shut. Upon opening, the bathroom door immediately slams into the toilet. I shimmy in and hug the wall to close it. Then the room is black. Groping around, I find there's no light switch. I shimmy back between the toilet and wall and open the door and slip out. The bathroom switch is over by the entrance to the room. Slithering back in, I find the hot and cold taps are reversed and the sink rust-stained from a long-lived drip. And the place is apparently haunted.

"Careful of the paranormal," Brett warned me of the Lowe. "It's friendly, just lonely." From what I can see around town, I don't blame it.

With some trepidation—afraid that he might cancel—I call Matthew and confirm our meeting for tomorrow.

"I haven't heard from you. I was worried. Where are you?"

I tell him.

"What the fuck are you doing there? Get out of there."

Relieved we're still on track, I walk down deserted Main Street. After dark and under the collapsing marquee of the shuttered movie house, there's no denying the eerie quality about town. There's one restaurant, the Rio Bravo, Mexican fare. Resigned to an awful meal, I'm happily proven wrong.

Mid-taco, Seve finally calls back.

By now he's processed my barging in and treats it as nothing at all. I'm not sure if he knows I'm aware of how upset he was, but in classic guy fashion, since he's decided to simply move on, I do as well. He asks about my day, what I saw.

"Never been," he says. "Although I'd like to drive those back roads."

"I'll come get you, Seve."

He chuckles. "Soon, Little Buddy, soon."

Long ago there was a television sitcom called *Gilligan's Island*, about a group of shipwrecked castaways. The Skipper used to call Gilligan—his first mate—Little Buddy. Seve often used the nickname with me back in the day. I haven't heard it in years.

The mood of dread that's hung over me most of the day has lifted, and I drive a mile out of town, past Tudor's Biscuit World and McHappy's Donut Shoppe and the ubiquitous Dollar General to the Dairy Queen. I sit in the car in the corner of the dark parking lot in the cold and sip my chocolate shake, content. I wonder what people who live here do for fun. Watching car after car go through the drive-in to get their Misty Freeze, I realize I'm doing it.

Brookville, Ohio

Crossing over the Point Pleasant Bridge into Ohio, I am now in the Midwest and take up US Route 35. The sky is low, but the land here relaxes out to gently rolling farm country. A neatly rowed dirt field, waiting for spring. A blue grain silo. On the edge of a town, a gun supply store. Tate's Tree Service—"stump grinding a specialty." The Dollar General store. My mind drifts. More rolling hills. Dried corn stalks in dormant fields.

Something on my dash pings, breaking my road-induced trance. I've gone too far west. But the ping is telling me I need to fill my gas tank. On the outskirts of Brookville, Ohio, I turn into what can only be viewed as further deterioration of American culture and ingenuity—the combination gas station/convenience store/fast-food restaurant, which has become inescapable across the country. These overlit, soulless pods of supposed plenty have cancerized the environs of small and midsize towns, where other more locally nurturing options might prosper. That this is low hanging fruit for complaint does not make it any less true. I find such places depressing in their "convenience"—peddling alienation.

At the BP station, holding open the door for a large man laboring under the weight of a "family size fun pack" of M&M's and a gargantuan, plastic, refillable beaker of soda, I wonder if there is a worse idea than the sixty-four-ounce Big Gulp. I check my height against the tape measure attached to the door's frame—there to capture on video the height of any criminal looking for a quick score. Still disappointed I never approached six feet, I go in search of the bathroom.

Past the self-serve Slurpee machine (my childhood dream!), I find myself crossing an invisible line into Hardee's. It's here, in a hardbacked booth along the wall, sipping coffees, that I encounter Lew and Bobby.

Their faces sag with age, but their eyes are bright and offer up a direct gaze. Both men wear sweatshirts. Both wear baseball caps. Lew's is blue. Bobby's is fatigue-colored with a camouflage American flag patch on its crown. Even from a distance, the two emit a closeness. Thinking of my reticence with the group back in Elkins, I quickly push through my natural reserve before it can justify itself, and approach. The two readily tolerate a stranger's intrusion.

They grew up around the corner from each other in southern Ohio, not far from where they now live. Bobby was twelve when they met riding bicycles. Lew was fourteen. "When we grew up, kids were kids," Lew says, sipping his coffee. Both have been married twice—Lew for fifty-two years, Bobby for forty-nine. Both have two grown children. They went to the same college and worked on the ambulance squad. They were police officers, working together for a time. Each has had open-heart surgery. After retiring, both men went back to work, Lew for the volunteer fire department, Bobby keeping the books for the cemetery.

Lew and Bobby have an "unwritten policy" to get together at least once a week. "It's a stress reliever," Bobby says of their get-togethers. Both return home after a morning spent in the other's company in a "mellow" mood. If they haven't seen each other in a while, Lew's wife is quick to suggest he needs "some Bobby time."

"My wife is my soulmate," Bobby says, then elbows his friend. "But he knows where the bodies are buried."

"Yeah, we trash everything." Lew laughs. "He's my voice of reality. We've been together for sixty years. What keeps us together, we don't know. We're just two good ol' boys who like to do a job right, treat people right, we've got a work ethic and aren't afraid of challenges." He leans his shoulder into his friend. "Although he's a perfectionist to a fault."

"Yeah, and he always wanted to kick the door in." Bobby laughs. "I'd suggest turning the handle."

"That's true," Lew concedes.

There's something so seamless between these two that's alien to me.

"You two have any secrets from each other?" I ask.

Lew seems almost taken aback. "He's my psychiatrist. I'm his. I think I'm wacko till I talk to him. Then I know I'm normal."

"We're an open book," Bobby says. "I'm okay 'cause he's okay."

Are they aware they have something special?

Bobby nods gently. "There's a caveman mentality with a lot of men. 'I'm king of the hill. I don't need anyone.'"

"There's a lot of chest pounding," Lew agrees. "But that strategy doesn't age well. I tell you, there are a thousand people in my town and there are a lot of guys, a whole lot of guys, who just don't go out anymore. They're embarrassed to be seen as diminished, not what they once were. They become victims."

"Let me tell you something"—Bobby becomes animated—"without purpose you rot."

Lew goes on. "I want to get a bus and go around and pick up all these guys and take them to breakfast at Hardee's," Lew says.

"They need some fellowshipping. Seriously. There's a need in the population. I feel like I have a social and moral obligation."

"I imagine there's a lot of fear and ego involved," I say. "And no one wants to admit they're afraid."

"I think you're on to something there, Andrew," Lew says.

"It's an ego thing." Bobby nods. "A macho thing."

We sit in silence. Then Lew says, "We started telling each other 'I love you' last year." He leans in and starts to laugh. "And you know what that means, Andrew. You say 'I love you' to another man and you're queer."

"That's 'cause most men only think about sex," Bobby says.

Lew sits back and shakes his head. "I tell my kids I love them. Why can't I tell my best buddy that I love him?"

I can't help but think of Seve. Since we've begun speaking on the phone again on a regular basis, he'll conclude each call by telling me he loves me. I will rush farewells over his comment so as to make it seem like I didn't hear and hang up. I'm, of course, embarrassed by my childish actions. I constantly tell my wife and kids that I love them, but that phrase, when uttered by a man in such a circumstance, makes me quickly uncomfortable.

When I was a small child, I was terrified of my father's volatile temper. I never felt that he liked me. Yet he would often tell me he loved me. I was naturally expected to complete the exchange, "I love you, too." I grew increasingly uncomfortable with this, until, at around the age of ten I began to respond, "I hate this part. I love you too." My father always laughed at my amendment, but I knew it angered him. And that latent anger scared me. Yet I took satisfaction in this small bit of power I could claim with my reply. Add to this that it was the truth. I hated having to parrot back a phrase that to me felt insincere coming from someone who so often—because of his temper—behaved in a way toward us that felt the opposite of love. That such a parent–child dynamic should have such long tentacles and bleed over into my adult male friendships is what keeps psychiatry couches full—if that in fact is what's even at play here. Or maybe, like so many men, I just have issues of confusing love and intimacy with sex.

But Lew clearly has no such problem. "I used to wear this pink shirt with my suit. People would say, 'You must be secure in your manhood.'" He shakes his head and points between himself and his friend. "We know where we're at."

Bobby lowers his voice. "We haven't graduated to a good-night kiss."

The men laugh together. Something they do easily.

"But when it's time, we cry together too." Lew looks at Bobby. "When your parents died."

"And your brother."

These two know the value of what they have. "Our social circles are small. We know a lot of people, but"—Lew looks to his friend—"we have each other."

"We have so much in common, the two of us are one," Bobby concludes simply.

Lew nods. "We'll have to go at the same time, 'cause one couldn't live without the other. They'll just have to put one on ice till the other's ready."

There's a long history of the kind of platonic romance these two men share. One of the more famous examples is Abraham Lincoln's friendship with Joshua Speed. And while that relationship has been reexamined, with some concluding it was sexual, the bromances of the eighteenth and nineteenth century were often more demonstrative and affectionate and of a different nature than most male friendships of today.

Intimate expressions of fidelity and letters between men baring confidences were commonplace. Alexander Hamilton, in a letter to fellow soldier John Laurens in 1779, wrote, "I wish, my dear Laurens, it might be in my power, by action rather than words, to convince you that I love you... 'till you bade us Adieu, I hardly knew the value you had taught my heart to set upon you."

Add to this that physical interaction between men and women, until married, was largely restricted—men were freer with affection and physical contact toward one another.

But less than a hundred years later all that had changed. Gone were genteel sensibilities of the Gilded Age. By the time World War II concluded, the transformation of the image of the ideal American man had morphed into that of a macho, strong, and largely silent lone wolf. The conception of heterosexual friendship and intimacy that we accept today as normal has traveled a long distance from Lincoln's time, becoming profoundly more restricted in its expression.

I leave these two friends laughing as they refill their coffee. Then, avoiding the eight lanes of I-75 that can take a traveler from Michigan to Miami without making an exit, I head southeast on local Route 35, bypassing Cincinnati. Past pleasant farmland, then south onto Route 62, through the town of Hillsboro, under a grumpy sky spitting rain, a thought that's been playing along the edge of my mind starts to come clear. Two things that Lew said keep coming back to me—two seemingly disparate comments, yet they seem linked.

The first is that his and Bobby's friendship "keeps getting better," even after all these years. And the second is that Lew said he no longer had sex, something he mentioned twice. An obviously private admission, he volunteered it freely to a stranger without prompting or shame. That surrendering of potency, the relinquishing of such power, changes a man's place in the world. Especially someone whose work was defined by power—what's a more obvious example of male power and potency than being a cop?

So many men are defined by our relation to these qualities. Sexual conquests when we're young go a long way in establishing our sense of masculine identity in the world. Exerting power over others, achieving dominance, be it in sports, the bedroom, or the boardroom, is how so many men keep score, the yardstick by which we measure our lives a success. What happens when that power wanes?

There's a line in Arthur Miller's classic play centered on this theme of diminishing male potency, *Death of a Salesman*—"Life is a casting off," Linda Loman counsels her despairing husband, who isn't ready to relinquish the speck of power he has.

This is what Lew was referring to when he spoke of the men in his town who he said felt diminished, the men he wanted to round up and take to breakfast. Something has to fill that cavernous space left by the loss of that self-defining potency, or else what is a man left with but anger and resentment?

But Lew and Bobby appear to understand something that has given them clarity, peace, and a gentleness that I found almost unsettling. With the loss of potency has come an acceptance that has fostered intimacy and openness. The relinquishing of the slavish obligation to serve a receding potency has created room for their friendship to "keep getting better."

Paris, Kentucky

The rain on Route 62 has picked up, and I flip on my wipers for the first time. They begin to snap hard. In a few minutes the wiper on my driver side begins to fling itself off the edge of the car with each pass, growing wilder and more erratic with every swipe. I'm afraid it will snap off. I turn the wipers off, but the rain comes down hard and I turn them on again. Instantly the wiper is hurling itself off the car with violence. I'm forced to pull over and wait out the deluge. I detour to Cincinnati airport to swap out my blue Chevy Malibu for a nearly identical red one. In a move that is surprisingly seamless, I'm back on the road in less than an hour.

In gloomy Aberdeen, I turn onto Simon Keaton Memorial Bridge over the Ohio River and I'm back in the South, in Kentucky. Route 68 takes me forty miles down the road to Paris. Founded in 1790 and home to ten thousand, it boasts a handsome downtown that recently joined the ranks of Paris, Tennessee; Paris, Michigan; Paris, Mississippi; Paris, Texas; Las Vegas; and Epcot Center in Florida—not to mention Prague, Bolivia, New Zealand, and of course, France—with an Eiffel Tower of its own. This one rises from a parking lot on the corner of Eighth Street and Main. While measuring a humble twenty-five feet high, for some reason I'm compelled to snap a dozen photos of the diminutive reproduction.

Just down the block, a bronze statue of favorite four-legged son, Secretariat, presides over the small park bearing his name. A three-story mural of the colt in his blue-and-white Kentucky Derby winning silks is painted on an adjacent brick wall. The legendary Triple Crown winner retired to stud at nearby Claiborne Farms, solidifying Paris's place as a horse breeding mecca.

It was my father who introduced me to Secretariat when I was ten. Not a horseracing fan that I was aware of, he nonetheless sat me down in front of the television for the Kentucky Derby, which Secretariat won handily. Then again a few weeks later for the Preakness and finally the Belmont Stakes. The great horse had by now captured the attention of not only my father and me, but the nation. Secretariat seemed to revive the confidence of a country that had lost its way, first with Vietnam and now with something starting to be called Watergate. The horse was big and brash and felt decidedly American.

I sat beside my father as Chic Anderson called the race on TV in awed disbelief, his voice bellowing with wonder, "He's moving like a tremendous machine! Secretariat by twelve! Secretariat by fourteen lengths…!" The champion would go on to win the Belmont by thirty-one lengths. He set track records in all three Triple Crown races that still stand, fifty years on.

As Secretariat crossed the line, my father and I leaped into the air and embraced. I was as thrilled by the win as I was to be, for a moment at least, in my father's favor. We were not the first men (if you can call a ten-year-old boy a man) brought together by sports.

Just up the block from the bronze stallion, the soda fountain of Lili's Coffee Shop occupies one wall of a vast room crammed with bric-a-brac, Ardery's Antiques. After a hot chocolate at the counter, I'm wandering through used furniture, mismatched china on doilies, porcelain dolls, brass lamps, trinkets of all variety, when I'm brought up short by an unusual photograph hanging high up on the wall above the door. It's black-and-white, perhaps seven feet long by just one foot high. On the far right of the shot is a galloping thoroughbred, behind him is a vast expanse of empty racetrack, and on the left edge of the picture is the nearest horse. The photo captures Secretariat crossing the wire so far out in front in that famous Belmont Stakes race my father and I cheered on.

"Great photo, isn't it?" says the woman who served my hot chocolate, Nancy, the manager at Lili's. She's suddenly standing by my side.

"If my father were alive, I'd get it for him," I say softly.

Nancy knows enough to leave that comment alone. "Want to meet the vet who saved him?"

"Huh?"

"Dr. Copelan, he saved Secretariat right before the Derby. He's at the table in the back, with those other fellas. They're here every Tuesday. I'll introduce you."

I had noticed the group of four middle-aged and elderly men, empty coffee cups on the table in front of them, chatting. They're only too eager to have some fresh blood join their round table. Dr. Copelan, now ninety-one, is diminutive and bald with thick glasses and a gutter mouth. He also needs little prompting to share the famous story.

"Go on, Doc. Tell him," says Beau Lane, a burly, silver-haired horseman sporting a massive belt buckle and a leather vest that he probably wears 360 days a year. When he elbows the tiny man beside him, I half expect the good doctor to be flung out of his chair across the room.

"Shit, he doesn't want to hear it," the doctor says, but then launches in before I can assure him that I do.

Secretariat, the definitive favorite going into the Kentucky Derby, had shockingly lost a race just a few weeks earlier. No one knew why. So, with just over a week before the big one, Dr. Copelan had been asked to take a look at the stallion. He approached stall 42 at Churchill Downs and grabbed Secretariat's halter. Copelan then went to stroke the colt's muzzle.

"That son of a bitch reared back and almost smashed his Goddamn nose on the upper stall. I suspected instantly what it was. Eventually, he let me take a look, and I was right, that poor bastard had a nasty abscess on the inside of his upper lip. I told Shorty—"

"Shorty?" I interject.

"The groom," the doctor snaps like I'm an idiot.

"His name was Eddie Sweet," the wiry Black man missing several teeth and sitting at the end of the table explains patiently. This is Randy, Copelan's long-time assistant and friend. "He looked after the horses in the barn."

"A good groom," Copelan says. "But he could get distracted by a pretty face."

"Go on, Doc," Beau redirects his friend. "What did you tell Shorty?"

They've all heard the story a million times. They all clearly enjoy it, but what they really appear to appreciate is how much their friend relishes telling it—seeing him come alive under its spell.

"I said, 'Shorty, now you listen here. You do exactly what I say, damn it. No shortcuts.' And he did, thank God."

"But tell him what you told him, Doc," Bob Clark, a thoughtful man in a plaid shirt sitting beside me, reminds the doctor.

"Oh yeah," Copelan says. "Well…" He sits up and rubs his hands together.

Everyone at the table is smiling at the old man.

"I told him, 'You listen to me, you son of a bitch. You put a hot Turkish compress on that lip for seven minutes of every hour of the day. Seven minutes, no more, no less. Every hour. I'll be back tomorrow.' I hoped that would do the trick, 'cause I sure as hell did not want to have to lance that ornery bastard, especially with no anesthesia, since it was so close to the Derby and he couldn't have those drugs in him and race."

"Did you think they were gonna have to scratch him?" Bob cues Copelan.

"Not if I had anything to say about it. But it was sure looking that way. Every morning I'd go right to his stall first. I kept hoping I'd hear Shorty call out to me good news when I arrived, but every morning he'd just mumble 'Mornin' Doc.' It wasn't looking good. Then just four days before the Derby, Shorty said, 'Doc, I think that abscess might have drained.' And God damn it, it had. I flushed it out, big necrotic plug popped out, and you know the rest."

The doctor sits back, triumphant in his retelling. The table beams. I've been brought into the fold.

"Now, what about you, young fella?" Copelan asks me.

"Well"—I shift under the table's gaze—"I did drag a dead body around in a movie, so I guess we're kind of even." In my youth I appeared in a ridiculous black comedy called *Weekend at Bernie's* that has achieved a kind of cult status.

"I saw that!" Bob says. "Hysterical."

"Any movies with horses?" the doctor asks me.

I spare the men any mention of my lone cowboy movie, and the table rallies around equestrian films. "When Phar Lap goes up that hill, I still get tears rolling down my cheeks," Beau says, ignoring the ringing phone in the pocket of his leather vest.

They talk with knowledge and admiration of the work of Sam Shepard, who lived in nearby Midway. But what impressed them most about the playwright and movie star was his roping ability.

Beau's phone rings for the second time.

"Jesus, Beau, you've only got two friends and we're both here. Who could be calling you?" Bob teases.

Beau looks to me. "You know Bob sold me some junk piece of art? I don't know why I still talk to him." The table laughs. The two friends happily bicker back and forth on the differing details of the transaction that began their friendship—the truth seems to have been willfully cast aside long ago.

Bob puts a hand on my shoulder. "We don't call ourselves the Liar's Club for nothing."

Then Beau's tone turns serious. "Bob is the premier equestrian artist in the world, Andrew," he says with pride, squinting at his friend with affection.

Conversation around the table splinters, and Bob leans over to me. "Beau brought me into the group when I moved to town several years ago. It was like the papal blessing. He's got twenty years on me, but I look upon him the same way I would look upon my dad if he were still here." Bob glances at his friend across the table. "He's a man of his word, salt of the earth. Tuesdays with these guys is the highlight of my week. Theirs too. Something pretty big would have to be happening to miss this."

I wonder aloud what specifically it is about this group.

"If laughing is good for your health, we are all in very good health," Beau says by way of explanation.

"I'll never need a psychiatrist with this group," Bob says. "I've got three of them right here."

Doc pushes his chair back to go to the bathroom. Randy offers a hand and the good doctor slaps him away. Bob leans close again. "And the thing is, Andrew," he says softly, as if not wanting to embarrass himself or the rest of the group, "we show up for each other. It is absolutely the most important ingredient. If someone is going through something, they're being tested in some way, you show up for them and the relationship gets stronger. If something happens to someone in this core, I'm there. And shame on you if you're not there when they need you."

"What lies are you telling over there?" Beau cuts in.

"None of your business, old man," Bob shoots back.

As the gathering breaks up, we all bunch together and photos are taken and shared and Doc squeezes my arm. "You come back next Tuesday, Andrew. You're welcome here."

Heading out of town, I see a small sign and make a quick left onto Winchester Road. Down a swale and over the railroad tracks, Claiborne Farm is just a mile up the road. It's here that Secretariat is buried beneath a regal headstone.

A "No Trespassing" sign is mounted on the stone pillar that supports an open iron gate. Beneath it another sign reads, "By Appointment Only," while a third informs any interloper that the entire property is under twenty-four-hour surveillance. Undeterred, I turn into the long drive. Rolling green hills are bound by four-rail fences. There are distant outbuildings. The word "majestic" would not be out of context here. The first building I come upon has a sign reading "Visitor Center." I pull into the large and empty lot. Another sign lists the opening hours as 9:30–12:30. It's late in the afternoon. As I peer into the dark window, I can see in its reflection that a white SUV has quietly pulled into the far end of the lot and idles, exhaust rising from its tailpipe.

I don't know exactly what I was looking for here, perhaps just to stand over Secretariat's grave for a moment—my father would have liked that. I return to my car and pass the idling SUV with tinted windows, the word "Police" stenciled on its side. Through the gate, I make my way back toward town. The SUV follows close behind, very close. I turn onto Main Street and pass the Eiffel Tower, the trooper still on my heels. If I hit the brakes quickly, he will rear-end me. Only when I've cleared town and am back in open country does the tailgating cop pull a sharp U-turn and head back to town. Maybe I should have told him I'm a friend of Doc Copelan.

Lexington, Kentucky

We were night shooting. I'd arrived to work shortly before dusk in my recently purchased 1967 Camaro convertible. It was 1985 and I was twenty-two and on the cusp of becoming a movie star. The scene we were shooting was set at a nightclub in West Hollywood, standing in for suburban Illinois. As is often the case in movie making, I had hours to kill before I was needed.

Sitting on the steps of my dressing trailer, I was taking in the evening, watching crew and actors come and go.

"Hey!" a voice called.

A tall and thin man with dark eyes and black hair came walking across the parking lot as night fell. Matthew was on set visiting the director and saw me killing time. He and I had acted in a movie together a year earlier. We didn't know each other well—we hadn't really connected then—but now we did.

Matthew and I became fast friends. As a young actor I feared Los Angeles and dreaded my time there. An insecure kid, I felt under scrutiny, exposed, always "on." I was becoming a public figure. People began to come at me, wanting, watching, judging. Matthew desired nothing from me but my friendship. We drank and shot pool at Barney's Beanery on Santa Monica Boulevard. We played golf in Griffith Park. We took impulsive runs up the California coast. We chased girls. Mostly we laughed. His friendship felt like a life raft while I was tossed amid a school of Hollywood barracuda.

As I was finishing the movie, I decided to drive my new Camaro back home to New York. Matthew planned to join me for the trip cross-country—"I should go see Betty anyway," he said. Matthew's mother was an active part of his life and came out to visit him often. And since I was her son's friend, and she was a classic Jewish mother, Betty offered me no choice and pulled me under her wing as well. I playfully called her "Ma."

On the day we were to leave LA, work came up for Matthew and he had to cancel. I decided to go alone. I'm not sure how far I thought I'd get, but I made it to Las Vegas, five hours east. Three days later I was still holed up at the Tropicana. I'd lost all my money for the trip home. (Amex had wisely declined my application for a credit card.) I called my friend.

"Sport," I croaked into the phone. "You gotta come get me."

Matthew flew in and dragged me out of the hotel. The valet brought my red convertible around, and as he did, I remembered an uncashed check in the car's glove compartment—a few hundred dollars for living expenses I'd received from the movie.

"Let's go back in!" I cried.

"No." Matthew was firm.

"Sport, it's a sign from the universe."

"You're drunk."

"Please!" I begged. He hesitated. I could see him wavering. "Let's flip a coin," I said. "Heads we leave. Tails we go back in."

My friend stared at me. "I'm calling it."

"Fine."

I tossed the coin.

"Heads," Matthew said.

The coin landed on the parking lot and rolled beneath the car. I crawled under. "Tails," I screamed from below the transmission.

The hotel was eager to cash my check from Paramount Pictures, and we sat down side by side at the blackjack table. In less than a half hour we won back all I'd lost and more. Matthew grabbed me by the scruff of my neck. The car was still waiting by the front door of the casino.

"I'm driving," he said, and got behind the wheel.

With the top down, I leaned my head back and looked up into the stars while a hot desert wind whipped. We sang along to Dire Straits' "Money for Nothing" over and over back to Los Angeles. I shipped the car home.

For a time, I kept a room at Matthew's bungalow. I tossed a mattress on the floor of his spare bedroom and considered it decorated. It was far from the glamorous pad of a young Hollywood up-and-comer, but it felt safe—and fun. Only twice did Matthew scold me about being such a fucking slob. He made no judgment regarding my show biz reticence but would occasionally implore me to "Go to the fucking party, Mr. Hermit. You might even get laid."

Matthew eventually grew disenchanted with Los Angeles and show business and left. It was a step I admired—many complain, few make the split. He moved east to North Carolina to pursue his passion—sportscasting. I saw less of him. Then I got a call.

"Sport," Matthew said over the line. "I'm getting married."

"I didn't know you had a girlfriend," I replied.

He'd met a woman. There was going to be a baby. The wedding would be in Louisville, Kentucky, her hometown.

"I'm coming," I said.

"No, don't," Matthew said. "It's not going to be a big deal. We're just doing it at this house. No one is coming."

"Just tell me when it is and give me the address," I said and got on a plane.

His wife's family filled the generous living room of a grand Richardson Romanesque mansion rented for the occasion. Matthew's bride came down the stairs while he waited at the landing to receive her. I felt for my friend that day, the "Jew from Long Island" marrying into a family of strict Southern Baptist Evangelicals he had just met. Standing on that landing, he seemed very alone. Yet Matthew survived and raised two children in Kentucky and only recently got divorced.

As with Seve, whenever we'd talk on the phone it was as if no time had passed. We'd make plans to get together, a golfing trip, Ireland, Vegas. Nothing ever came of it.

My police escort out of Paris having lost interest, I pass large houses with imposing porticos and pillars set far back from the road. The sun sneaks through robust clouds, slashing God's light down.

By the time I've found my way to Matthew's modest suburban Lexington neighborhood, the clouds and drizzle have returned. I ease onto a small cul-de-sac and there he is, still tall, still thin, wearing a black baseball cap and walking a black, wiry mixed breed straining at his leash down the hill. I park in front of his house.

"Blue pooped," he calls out by way of greeting. "My day is made."

"He's black," I say, climbing out of the car, stating the obvious but questioning the name.

"He has one blue eye," Matthew explains as he gets closer.

"Shouldn't you have called him Bowie?"

"Not in Kentucky."

We embrace.

Once inside his small split-level, we gravitate to the kitchen. I lean against the counter as he boils me some water for the tea bag I produce from my pocket.

"Tea?"

I shrug.

"Boy, times change. I remember when you'd ask me to pour vodka in that cup."

He begins to parse out some pills.

"What are you taking there, Sport?" I ask.

"This one is for my cholesterol. This one I've been taking since my heart attack. This—"

"You had a heart attack?" I shriek. "When?"

"Thirteen years ago." Matthew's ex-wife came home from work one night, looked at her husband and called 911. Within an hour he had a stent implanted to clear the hundred-percent blockage of his artery.

"How the fuck did I not know you had a heart attack?" I say, shaking my head. "I know I've been a negligent friend, but that's kind of a big one to miss."

"Well, I see you every day," Matthew says. "I got a picture of us from your and Carol's wedding on the dresser in my room." Matthew was the best man at my first wedding.

"That picture has lasted longer than the marriage did." I shrug.

"How is Carol?" he asks after my former wife, and chats about her with affection. Then talk turns to kids. "I remember one time, after Everett was born, he had colic and wouldn't stop crying. I called you in the middle of the night and said I was going to kill him. You told me about the time you wanted to climb up to the roof and throw Sam off 'cause he wouldn't stop crying. I'm telling you, that saved me. That really helped."

"I'm not sure either one of us would win father of the year for that one."

Then we're discussing the end of his marriage.

"Her clothes are still in the closet."

"How long has it been again?" I ask.

"A year."

I raise my eyebrows.

"Hey, no judgment," he says.

I hold my hands up in surrender.

"I still pay her phone bill for God's sake," he says.

"I understand that guilt," I say.

"Yeah, but..." He shakes his head.

We try, but neither of us can remember the last time we saw each other. "I've lived here in Lexington for fourteen years, and it certainly hasn't been in that time." In fairness to myself, Matthew has been just as lax as me. Like me, his marriage and kids and work consumed him, with little time or resources left over. Or so our excuse goes.

Over time my tolerance for rejection has waned—my skin has gotten thinner, not thicker. Consequently, I vowed some time ago that I would no longer put myself in a position to be as cavalierly dismissed as is required of an actor. The result being that I've walked away from acting for the most part. Yet occasionally something comes up that catches my attention.

I was asked to audition for a movie project, the type of part I'd never done. I was intrigued, and the following morning ask Matthew to play the scene with me and make a tape in his kitchen to show the director. There are very few people with whom I'd feel comfortable enough to do such a thing. But back in the day, Matthew and I did several movies together. Acting was how we met. It's how we used to identify and locate ourselves. It's something bone deep for both of us (even though neither of us does it much anymore). I set up my phone on his kitchen table and feel a stab of shame.

Maybe it's simply that my vanity has kicked in because I'm about to be filmed, or maybe it has something to do with how exposed I feel when I act, or perhaps it's because my friend used to do this with me so many years ago, when we were young and felt an invincibility that has long since faded. Whatever the reason, I turn to my friend.

"I'm really embarrassed to have gotten old, for you to see me old."

Matthew looks at me, considers my face, then shrugs.

I feel received by that shrug, liberated by it, emboldened by it.

We spend the next half hour filming and refining the scene. It's fun. The way acting used to be.

We then drive into downtown Lexington, where Matthew has a live pregame and postgame basketball show to do, broadcast from the corner of a large and bustling sports bar.

On the way I mention a roadside sign I saw while driving down. The Hatfield and McCoy Trail. The legendary feud between the two families was something that fascinated me as a child. "I didn't know the houses still existed. Did you? There's this whole driving tour you can do to all the sites where they shot each other and all of it."

"So?" My friend is clearly not interested.

"Let's go tomorrow. Where's Pikeville?"

"I can't. It's Pike*vul*."

"Huh?"

"It's pronounced Pikevul, not Pikeville."

"See? This is why I need you. I might get a whoopin' if I go alone."

"If I'm your protection in rural Kentucky, God help you."

"We'll be home by dinner," I promise.

"Unless we get a whoopin'."

The next morning we're having breakfast at a diner called Wild Eggs, in the strip mall around the corner from his home. My friend has not budged in his refusal to drive across the state to the West Virginia border.

"Look. It's God's cruel joke that he put me here in the first place. Punishment for all I did. No way am I chasing the ghosts of some fucking hicks to the middle of bumfuck nowhere."

"I'll see you for dinner," I say, pouring more syrup on my pancakes.

Matthew lifts his coffee to his lips and mutters, "Maybe."

Pikeville, Kentucky

The truth is, Matthew's right. I am chasing a ghost. As a boy of nine I had a best friend named Sean. He lived directly across the street. Sean's family moved around a lot and they didn't stay long, but while they were there, Sean and I were inseparable. One day, after seeing something on television, Sean became obsessed with the Hatfields and the McCoys. His preoccupation fueled mine, and we learned all we could about the infamous feud that has long been a metonym for any bitter rivals.

The more prosperous Hatfields lived on the West Virginia side of the Tug Fork of the Big Sandy River, while the McCoys lived primarily on the Kentucky side. The origins of dispute are varied and confusing, but suffice to say it involved a pig, property, and moonshine. The warring lasted for nearly thirty years after the Civil War, with up to eighteen family members losing their lives, depending on whose account is to be believed.

I hadn't thought about Sean much in recent years, but the road sign I'd passed snapped me back to the afternoon spent at my house looking through the World Book Encyclopedia and then across the street at his, scanning his father's stack of *National Geographic*s hoping for any details of the family feud. It was soon after this that Sean's family moved away suddenly. I never got a chance to say goodbye and never saw him again. I came home from school and they were gone. Sean was my first best friend.

Maybe I'm grasping for a touchstone or looking to get some kind of closure for a long-ago loss, but when Matthew goes off to do his radio show I head east.

The sky is slate gray, the trees along the Mountain Parkway are mostly bare, abandoned birds' nests visible high in their branches. An hour east of Lexington, in Clay City, I pull off looking for some hot water for my tea. Nearly forty percent of the one thousand residents here live below the poverty line.[1]

There's not much going on in the way of street life. The fenced-in yard at the Happy Hearts Day Care, filled with overturned toys and a plastic slide, is empty and overgrown. There's no one about at the Church of God, nor the Clay City Baptist Church. A large auto graveyard filled with hundreds of rusting wrecks occupies an empty field across from M&S Pawn Shop. There's a DQ, but no other restaurants. There is no coffee shop.

I stop at the IGA supermarket, still looking for a cup of hot water. I'm the only customer in the place. Many of the white metal shelves are rusted at their edges and sparsely filled. Much of the produce appears wilted, and the prepared foods in hot plates were not cooked this morning. A lone young man is behind the register. He's tall, with pale skin and dark hair. He has a nose piercing. His name is Kent.

"Pretty quiet around here," I say, stating the obvious.

"It is," Kent confirms.

"You from here?"

"Yeah."

"What do people do for fun?"

Ken rolls his eyes—either in reaction to the obvious stupidity of my question or a comment on the dearth of options.

"Well, I guess there's the nature preserve."

"What do you do?"

"I go fishing in the river."

"The Red River?"

"You can go out to the lake, but I like the river. You never know what you're gonna git."

"What's in there?"

"Catfish, bluegill, longear sunfish, maybe muskellunge."

"What do you use for bait?"

"Different things. Worms. Boot-tail grubs. I got a spinner."

"I haven't seen too many people around. There much social life here?"

"Mmm." Kent considers this. "You gotta go out of the county for that."

"And friends?"

"My friends are my enemies," Kent says with the matter-of-fact delivery that characterizes all his comments.

I try not to be taken aback by his frankness. "Why are they your enemies?"

"They don't want me to do better'n them."

"Ah."

"Or they want my girl."

I nod, looking around again at the half-filled shelves of processed breads and cartons of soda cans stacked high.

"So, I keep my circle close," Kent explains.

"Makes sense," I say, because it seems I should say something.

Kent considers me. "You ask a lot of questions."

"Sorry."

"You new 'round here?"

"Just passing through."

"Lucky."

Although I fail to get any hot water for my tea, I drive off in better spirits. And there's some social science to explain why. In 1973, Stanford sociologist Mark Granovetter produced a seminal paper showing the import of brief conversations and contact with those outside our primary circle and how important they are in providing information and opportunity. He called them "weak ties." Further studies followed, all leading in one direction. Casual interactions, ordering a morning latte, talking with the gas station attendant, and even contact with people met only once, like the random supermarket chat I just had with Kent, can prove as helpful in reestablishing a sense of well-being and belonging as connecting with family or closer friends.[2]

Beyond the Daniel Boone National Forest is a massive works program blasting through desolate hills. The goal is to transform the Bert T. Combs Mountain Parkway from what has been labeled one of the country's "most feared" two-lane roads for its twists, mountain passes, and descents into a safer scenic wonder. It's difficult to see the need for such expansion today as I'm the only one on the road. Route 23 leads me south and then suddenly, after such rural pleasures, the last half dozen miles into Pikeville feel like one long strip mall.

My first stop is the end of the line. Dils Cemetery is located along the bypass road at the mouth of Chloe Creek. It covers a steep hill, replete with tilting and fading headstones, gnarled trees, and encroaching ground ivy. It's here that several of the McCoy family rest, including Randal, the patriarch, and his wife, Sara. While the couple occupy a position near the top of the hill, son Sam is buried down near the road just behind Dorsie's Dairy

Bar & Ice Cream Shop, deep in thicket. Maybe the feud was not just with the Hatfields.

A few blocks away, Randal's house is now Chirico's Restaurant, home to "authentic Italian cuisine." Leaving town, I drive deep along twisting and narrow roads, east. Following Blackberry Creek, I locate the log cabin where the fateful trial over the pig that may or may not have been stolen was held—and set so much hatred in motion. The cabin is locked up tight, the windows obscured. Then in Hardy, in the backyard of one very indulgent local resident, lies the well that supplied water to McCoys' homestead. It was here that a midnight raid by the Hatfields ended in multiple deaths and with the McCoys' home burned to the ground.

This has all begun to feel like a fool's errand, with each stop more fruitless than the last.

My friendship with Sean was real and meaningful, formed at an age when friendship meant independence and individuality—when the discovery of a kindred spirit was revelatory and easy. And because of grown-up issues and parental disregard, that friendship was severed abruptly. But the only thing at the bottom of McCoys' well is rancid-looking water. There's nothing here to reclaim.

I get in the car and head back toward Lexington.

Retracing my route past the strip malls and then heading east on 23, I wonder what the hell I'm doing, so far from home and my family. It felt important, but right now it's difficult to justify grinding west through the voluminous construction on the Mountain Parkway.

Then Seve calls. In a typical mood, Seve is actively gregarious, always positively focused—at least to the outside world—but today he's in a pensive mood. It takes some time, but eventually he comes to the point of his call, what he needed to share. "I feel like a failure," he says simply.

Feelings of failure are something I'll confess easily over coffee, but I've never heard my friend admit such a thing.

I take a breath, then—"Well, Severino, you called at a very auspicious moment," I pronounce with exaggerated grandiosity.

"Oh, no," Seve says, hearing my suddenly grandiose tone. "Here it comes."

"I just happened to be listening to the Joseph Conrad novel *Lord Jim*—"

"You're listening to Joseph Conrad?" Seve is incredulous.

"Yeah, dude. He's awesome. You should check him out. Anyway, there was just this scene where Marlow is trying to calm a woman, explain something about Jim to her, and he finally blurts out, 'Nobody, nobody is good enough.'"

That hangs in the air for a moment.

"So, you see, my friend," I conclude, "you're in good company."

And if that doesn't suffice, I begin a rant of my multiple failings and disappointments, including what a lousy parent and spouse I am, out here on the road searching for I don't even know what.

Seve laughs and in turn admits what set off his current mood. Our conversation rambles, he relaxes, my spirits rise, and my long slog back passes more quickly. After we hang up, the obvious occurs to me—Seve would not have made that call even a few months ago, before we began speaking on a regular basis again.

Suddenly a sign on my dash illuminates—"Maintenance— Tire Pressure." Knowing nothing about this car, or any car, I assume this means that one of my tires needs air. I pull over and literally kick all four tires. They seem sound to me. I get back on the road. For the first time in days the sun comes out—just in time for it to set.

At dinner in a downtown Lexington steakhouse, Matthew gloats only a little over my needless side trip. "Told ya."

"So, I got a better idea," I say.

"Uh-oh."

"Got an open mind?"

"What is it?"

"Are you breathing?"

"Get to the point."

"Graceland."

"No."

Matthew and I share a deep and abiding love for Elvis Presley. Years ago, he sent me a Christmas ornament, a golden bust of the King. To my wife's dismay, it crowns our tree every year. Although I've been twice, and Matthew once, we've always talked of going to Elvis's Memphis home together.

"It's only six hours away. Let's just go."

"I can't."

"You mean you won't."

"Andrew," he warns. End of discussion.

We talk taxes and money worries. It's a relief to share such perpetually overhanging anxieties. Then Matthew leans close.

"Vietnamese dong, Sport?"

"What?"

"Dong, the currency, is about to get revalued. It's going to explode."

"Meaning?"

"I bought two hundred dollars in dong. It'll be worth hundreds of thousands, any day now."

"Are you high?" I ask.

"Don't get any. See if I care."

We go back and forth like this. I've participated in get-rich-quick schemes in the past, and those ships have yet to come in, but who wants to be at sea if these dong actually do dock? I pull out my phone and buy a few hundred dollars' worth of the Vietnamese currency on eBay.

"Now just sit back and wait." Matthew smiles.

"But I still have to buy dinner tonight, right?"

"Absolutely."

Later we hurry into my car against the cold night and find a nearby gas station. Matthew pulls out a tire-pressure gauge.

"Look at you," I say, "Mr. Mechanic."

"That's me. You can keep this."

"You got me a present, Sport?"

Matthew screws up his face. "No, I had an extra."

We find some quarters, drop them in the air pump machine in the corner of the lot, and begin racing around like idiots, checking and filling the tires before our time runs out, giggling like nine-year-olds.

The following morning we're in our now usual booth at Wild Eggs. As we pay the bill, Matthew says, "Come out to my car for a sec."

Back in the eighties, Bruce Springsteen had a hit song, "Glory Days," about an older man looking back on his youth. As young men, Matthew and I listened to it often when driving around LA together. In one verse, the Boss sings about a woman—"Back in school she could turn all the boys' heads." Without fail, Matthew and I used to snap our heads to the left at this precise moment. Invariably, we'd laugh at our brilliance. This juvenile practice has continued ever since. Even through the decades when we didn't see each other and barely spoke. Out of the blue I would get a call, "Sport! Driving and just heard 'Glory Days,' turned my head in the car. Hope you did too."

Matthew leads me across the parking lot.

"Take a seat," he says, arriving at his car. I think I know what's coming.

We climb in, and he turns the ignition, a smirk on his face. He reaches for the radio dial, and now I'm sure I know what's coming. Cued up and waiting is "Back in school she could turn all the boys' heads."

Our own youth long gone, we turn in unison. Still juvenile, still brilliant.

Matthew has always had the ability to veer from playfulness to deep emotionality, often in an instant. And he does so now.

He looks at me with feeling. "So glad you came down, Sport. I've missed you. I love you, man."

We embrace outside the car, and my friend heads off to do his radio show. I watch him drive away and sit for a long while behind the wheel of my rental. Just sitting.

Eventually I turn on the radio. A man with conviction in his voice is shouting, "The army of heaven is at your disposal!"

And my phone rings. It's my wife, Dolores.

"Listen, it's Dad's birthday in a few days, and I thought I'd take the kids over to Dublin and surprise him," she says.

This kind of impulsivity is more the norm than the exception with my wife. Routine and predictability are anathema to her. It took me only a decade to get used to this.

"Okay."

"Where are you again?" Dolores asks.

"Kentucky."

"I don't even know where that is." My wife is from Ireland, and America beyond New York is a vast and vague mystery. "How's Matthew?"

"He's great."

"You sound good."

"Did you know he had a heart attack a while ago?"

"No. But you certainly should have."

"Tell me about it," I say. "It was so good to just hang out. Talk. And do stupid stuff."

"I'm glad. You don't do enough stupid stuff."

"I think I do a lot of stupid stuff."

"Oh, I know," Dolores says. "But not the kind of stupid stuff that helps prevent the truly stupid stuff."

As we've been talking, an idea has begun forming in my mind. Then, as she does too often, my wife reads my thoughts. "How far is your friend Eddie from Kentucky?" she asks.

"Texas? It's a little ways."

"Anyway, we're on a plane tonight."

"Well, have fun," I say.

We hang up, and I sit still a little longer. Suddenly there is nothing pulling me toward home. *Eddie... why not?* I call him.

"Come on down, brother!" he shouts over the phone. "I'm just working here, trying to finish this fucking building, but we can hang. Let me know what flight you're on. I'll pick you up."

"I think I'm driving," I say.

"Road trip. I love it!"

Eddie

Leipers Fork, Tennessee

It takes me several minutes and a couple of laps past Wild Eggs to find my way out of the suburban parking lot.

"Am I doing this?" I say to no one as I lower the window and cold wind rips through the car. My impulsive acts to see both Seve and then Matthew sprang from a feeling of desperation, fear that the last vestiges of my friendships were slipping through my fingers. But based on the complicated satisfactions of my visits to Seve, and the simple pleasure of spending time with Matthew, this decision to carry on toward Eddie feels different. It feels more declarative, an active commitment to friendship, to showing up, to legacy, to loyalty.

I turn south.

There's no avoiding I-75 for a while, until bucolic Berea. There, I sip tea under a cold sun and wander through the idyllic college campus surrounding the town square. In a trick of the mind that produces connections according to its own logic, something in the specific red of the bricks reminds me of my high school, which looked nothing like this.

The main takeaway from my school experience was that I wasn't very smart. That I wasn't interested in what was being offered, or that I didn't fit into the mold in which it was delivered, never factored into the equation. Were it not for the few friends I had who had been likewise discarded by the powers-that-be, I don't know how I would have made it through. Chief among those friends was Scott Farley.

Scott was bigger than me, and he lifted weights in his basement. During our frequent sleepovers we'd smoke too much pot. Scott possessed what I would look back on now as an unfocused anger. I was too sensitive for my own good. We were unlikely friends. One day Scott passed me in the hall at school. "Let's go get pizza," he whispered. "Where?" I murmured back. He jerked his head in a "follow me" gesture, and we snuck off campus and dropped onto the trail beside the Elizabeth River. It felt to me as exotic and remote as if we were going up the Congo. Keeping out of sight, we walked a half mile and emerged back onto the pavement, cut quickly across the street, then slipped into a small freestanding pizza joint. How Scott knew about this place I had no idea, but in what became a Friday ritual, we each ordered a slice and a Coke, then put our feet up to bask in our freedom.

I never would have dared this excursion alone, nor would that have been of any interest. It was the camaraderie in our clandestine action that was so satisfying. Over those weekly lunches with my friend, I felt as if the life I had secretly suspected was out there waiting for me might finally be beginning.

Leaving Berea, I pick up Route 461. Outside the town of Pulaski, a thirty-foot cross looms beside the road. Once on the Cumberland Parkway, a billboard advises me to "Trust Jesus Before It's Too Late!" Then another assures me "In the Beginning, God Created Life." To emphasize the point, beside the words is the drawing of a man/ape in the evolutionary process inside a red circle with a red line cutting diagonally across it. "Does this kind of advertising work?" I ask the empty car.

There's a T.J.Maxx ahead. I detour and buy a couple of cheap shirts, then cross into Tennessee, moving south and west. Past Nashville, I'm back in country, wealthy country. Gentleman farms and well-manicured estates with long drives leading to columned houses sit atop cascading hills. Chestnut horses dip graceful necks and nibble shining grass inside symmetrically fenced fields.

Leipers Fork, forty miles south of Nashville, is one of those idyllic villages that "tick the boxes." It has two-lane charm, historic buildings that have been discreetly and artistically restored, rustic farm-to-table restaurants, and at Fox & Locke, a music venue that attracts wannabes and world-class talent. It's a town aware of its success. At one trinket shop disguised as home decor, a T-shirt is prominently displayed with the phrase "Don't Californiaize my Leipers Fork." Judging from the amount of cosmetic surgery that's been performed on the face behind the counter, it's too late.

Just away from Old Hillsboro Street, things are humbler. With no motels in town, I'm looking for the Airbnb I just booked. Up a winding track, past an un-signposted intersection, a Confederate flag hangs from the low porch of a worn-out house. A rusting sedan, its tires gone, sits among long weeds out front. Two small dogs, one brown, one black, come tearing out. The dogs' barking might be ferocious if it weren't so yappy. I slam on the brakes, concerned with not running them over as they leap in front of my car and disappear under the grill. They're too small for me to see where they've gone. It's silent for a moment as I wait for the dogs to run off. The black one then springs up directly outside my open driver's window, growling and baring its pointed teeth inches from my face, startling the shit out of me.

I jump, then hit the gas—only half hoping they've scattered.

The next yard along the road has been more lovingly attended to—I make a right on the manicured gravel driveway. A blonde, in her thirties, with very white teeth and a sunny disposition, steps out of an aluminum structure. She's sipping from a can of Red Bull. Her East Tennessee accent sings. She shows me to my generically cozy one-room cabin, five feet away from an identical generically cozy one-room cabin—one of four such cubes. Stefanie is my Airbnb hostess for the evening. She's a Superhost.

"Two beers in the fridge, two waters. Coffee maker. Need anything else, just holler."

"No Red Bull?" I say, referring to the can in her hand.

"I got one in the house. You want one?"

"I was joking," I say.

Stefanie looks at me sideways. "Oh, funny." Then she indicates the can. "It's why I never got COVID."

I let that homespun logic pass.

"Is there a key?" I ask.

Stefanie points to one in a basket beside the door.

"Do I need it?"

"We don't lock our door."

"Okay, then," I say, and leave the key untouched.

"Everyone in these parts is very well armed. Everyone knows that, so people don't just go wandering up to other folks' houses."

"Are you well armed?"

"I'm a Southern girl." She smiles, words dripping like flowered honey. "I'm not afraid to be alone out here."

"Well," I confess, "I am not well armed."

"Don't you worry, darlin'," she purrs. "I've got lots of friends."

"Good to have a friend." I nod.

Stefanie leans in. "Best friend in the world," she whispers. It's not entirely clear if she's referring to herself or her arsenal.

Then Stefanie spins, blond hair flying as she does, and calls over her shoulder, "I'm going into town. Y'all need anything?"

I smile, shake my head, and lock my cabin door.

Thursday is open mic night at Fox & Locke, and the place is packed. The stage is by the door, in front of a large window onto the street. The ceiling is low. A giant American flag hangs. The bar is tucked into a back corner, tables fill the rest. The MC for the evening relishes the sound of his own voice and asks for a hand for the military, and then another hand, then a third. The first performer does a credible George Strait cover. The second begins by telling the assembled that she's a believer. She sings two Christian originals. The crowd is warm and generous. Standing by the bar, I fall into conversation with a man named Jason—he moved to town from LA and makes his living as a real estate photographer. Jason came for the Southern hospitality and because "I can shoot my guns out the back door. Can't do that in the Valley."

"Not twice," I suggest.

Two bros around thirty approach. They recognize me from movies I've done. They've had a few beers and are effusive in their affection, but what they're even more compelled to express is how important movies in general are to their lives. "Our friendship was formed because of movies," the tall one, Mark, shouts over the music.

Tim, shorter and rounder, nods violently. "That's totally how we bond. It's because of movies that we're friends."

And it's through movies that the two communicate their emotions, comparing them to what certain characters are going through in a given movie. *The Hangover* and *I Love You, Man* feature prominently in the analysis of their feelings.

"Which one of you is Paul Rudd? The character who has no male friends?" I ask.

"Who do you think, man?" Tim asks.

"You?" I say, taking a guess.

"How did you know!?"

Mark enthuses how *Interstellar* relates to their lives, their friendship. "The sacrifices you make for people. Your dreams and purpose, separating you from everything. You know what I mean?"

I have to confess to Mark that I don't. "I never saw *Interstellar*."

"What?!" Tim steps back, aghast.

Mark tries to salvage some respect for me, imploring, "But you can understand what we're saying, right?"

It's important to them that I, someone who has been in movies, appreciate how vital the movies are to their bond.

"Everything in our lives, man, we relate to movies and each other," Tim promises me. "Remember in *Superbad*, those two best friends? That's us."

While alcohol may be fueling some of Tim and Mark's fervor, their passion speaks to something larger. Through movies—as with all art forms—people find identification, that identification fosters connection, and through that connection, we thrive. I assure my two new friends that I understand their passion—and share it.

Mark grabs my arm. "Just promise me you'll watch *Interstellar*. It's important."

Tupelo, Mississippi

Not interested in being told by my phone where to go or on what roads to drive, back in Harpers Ferry, West Virginia, I bought an oversize Rand McNally Road Atlas of the fifty states. A Luddite who enjoys poring over a map, imagining the lines on a page coming to life, wondering about the spaces in between, I thought it might keep me company for my few days on the road to Matthew. It's since proved very useful. Bulky and beginning now to get tattered along the edges, it's already been my dining companion more than a few times. "Wow," one waitress commented upon seeing me hunched over and awkwardly flipping between states, salt and pepper shakers pushed to the edge of the table to accommodate the map's size. "Haven't seen one of those in a long time."

I took silent pride in her comment as well as comfort in looking over and seeing the book beside me on the front seat across the miles. It's started to feel like a friend.

This morning I'm woken by an idea and reach for my cumbersome companion. I flip from Tennessee on page 186 to page 108.

Since I couldn't get Matthew to accompany me to Graceland, it would be only a slight detour on my way to Eddie to visit Elvis's birthplace in Tupelo, Mississippi, instead.

The Natchez Trace Parkway can take me right there. Tracking the original Native American route that evolved from a bison game trail, the path was used by European settlers as a thoroughfare between the Mississippi River and Cumberland plateau. Along its 444-mile route, simple inns sprang up to support travelers.

Today, sticking close to the old footpath, the parkway is by far the most bucolic, peaceful, pleasurable drive I've encountered in America. No signs, no advertising, no buildings or towns. Unlike every other road, whose function is merely a means to an end, the Natchez Trace Parkway comes close to being the event itself. And it allows my mind the space to begin making some sense of what's happening out here on the road.

By grinding miles across the country, I am honoring these friendships and my commitment to them—maybe even earning them back. But something else is also starting to register. I'm introducing myself to an America I thought I knew—the complicated and conflicted foundation that holds us and dictates so much of who we are and how we relate. I am of this place, this country. It is a part of me, of who I am. And it affects my relationships. By driving, I'm placing myself in a context, actively attaching to the legacy of imperfect interconnectedness. Consequently, it's of value to attempt, if not a thorough understanding—which would be impossible—at least an intimate exposure to it.

So serene, uncrowded, and elegantly laid into the land is the Natchez Trace Parkway that I am sorry to arrive in Tupelo, three carefree hours and 170 miles later. Then, like a homing pigeon, I turn off and proceed beneath the overpass of I-45, past the Dairy Kream, and make a left on Elvis Presley Drive.

Whereas Graceland is a mansion on the hill, the symbol of Elvis's success and excess, complete with jungle room and all the attendant silliness and sadness, his birthplace is a simpler shrine. It receives a fraction of the visitors heading to Memphis.

The bullet points of the Elvis legend are well known. Born into aching poverty. A nineteen-year-old truck driver walks into Sun Studios. The gyrations. The screaming girls. *The Ed Sullivan Show*. But it's almost impossible for us now to understand the impact Elvis had on the world. He not only changed what music was, but he redefined what celebrity meant and altered how stardom was embodied—a lot to place on the shoulders of a naïve country boy.

It quickly became impossible for Elvis to go anywhere and not be swarmed by dangerous crowds. When he wanted to see a movie, he had to rent out the theater. He loved to ride the Zippin Pippin roller coaster at Libertyland Amusement Park but had to close the place down to do so. Fame has many enticements, but it is among the most confining of experiences. By his twenty-first birthday, Elvis was isolated from society. In time that isolation would prove too much for even a king to survive.

The story of Elvis's rise becomes even more fantastical with one look at how his life began.

I arrive late in the afternoon. The first thing I notice, down close to the road, is the two-room shotgun shack where Elvis was born—built by his father, Vernon, for $180 (which he borrowed). There is no bathroom. The entire home, with original icebox and stove, takes seconds to view. The Assembly of God Pentecostal church, where the family attended services, has been relocated to the premises from a few hundred yards down the hill, and I'm late for the day's final presentation in the chapel.

I slip into the last of four rows just as the doors lock behind me. Three screens are lowered, one in front and one on either side, offering front and profile views—a primitive 2D version of 3D.

A video reenactment of what church was like in the early 1940s begins to roll. Barbara, the tour guide, offers up live commentary to accompany the film. "Life was hard, and church was all they had," she calls over the music. The people on the screen begin to sing, and Barbara sings along, clapping her hands, creating a kind of homemade, multimedia, immersive experience. A small boy in the role of Elvis on-screen gets up to sing what was his first public performance, "Jesus Loves Me." "This really happened," Barbara shouts with excitement. "Of course, the black hair came later, once Elvis saw Tony Curtis."

With the presentation over, Barbara, a retired English teacher from "out in bootleg country," confesses that "the Beatles were more my thing. But I've made friends from all over the world working here. Where else in Mississippi can I do that?"

Like many highly successful people who are self-taught, Elvis had a singular perspective and shrewd powers of observation. On the topic of friendship, he once noted, "Friends are people you can talk to, without words when you have to." And he surrounded himself with buddies from youth that he felt he could trust—what became known as the Memphis Mafia.

Just down the road is Johnny's Drive In BBQ. There's a photo on the wall of young Elvis seated in a booth, wearing his crooked grin. The waitress takes a shot of me in the same booth, attempting the famous sneer. Then it's on to Tupelo Hardware Co., where Elvis's mother, Gladys, bought her eleven-year-old son his first guitar.

My entire tour, while clearly silly, feels genuine, intimate. Everyone I encounter is engaged by my interest and shares in my passion. I promise myself I'll return with Matthew.

I pass the evening in the Blue Canoe, a roadhouse out on North Gloster Street, waiting for the band to start. My waitress, Kat, is the star of the room—greeting patrons as old friends, doling out hugs, sharing laughing asides with coworkers. We chat at length while she ignores her tables or charms others to handle them.

"You got a lot of friends here," I observe.

"Friends?" Kat raises an eyebrow. "Lot of acquaintances, but friends?" She shrugs.

"I understand," I say.

"It's lonely out there," Kat says, "so I keep busy."

I give up waiting on the band and overtip Kat on my way out. I feel for Kat but admire her candor—how easily she acknowledges her loneliness. Perhaps because women typically deal more readily in the realm of emotions than men, it's not such a big deal to admit. But as I'm beginning to see out on the road in America, from the most worshipped young singer in the world to my charming waitress, loneliness seeps.

Tupelo, Mississippi
Part 2

The following morning, I step out onto a deserted Main Street. The air is moist and warm. For no reason, I turn left. In short order I come upon the open green space of Fairpark, in the heart of downtown Tupelo. There stands a life-size statue of the favorite son. I slap the bronze Elvis's outstretched hand and keep walking. One block east I take a seat in the window at D'Cracked Egg.

The tables in the simple room are set wide apart. A young Indian woman covered in tattoos and plentiful piercings comes to take my order. She recommends the French toast. My tabletop is sticky.

The place is quiet on this Saturday morning, save for two older and elegantly dressed Black women eating in the corner. And at a large table along a brick wall, ten white men are gathered. They range in age—a few in their early twenties, many are middle-aged, a couple are older. All are dressed casually in plaids or sweatshirts. They're all focused on one of the younger men at the end of the table. He's talking quietly, his eyes looking at no one, his leg bouncing under the table. When the young man runs out of steam, a heavyset man at the center of the table speaks for the benefit of all.

"The devil speaks to some of the young, there's no denying. Remember, the devil is a master, and whichever way you want to go, he's willing to take you. But," the man goes on, "one stumble does not change your direction. Don't forget that. We don't want to be too pious about all this." He has the full attention of all assembled and speaks now to the young man directly. "You're moving in the right direction. You turn and the Lord's gonna be there. The mercy of God is upon you."

The young man nods. Others around the table nod as well.

The leader reassures the young man a bit more, talking about fellowship and brotherhood, then asks, "Cut a long story short, how do you feel?"

All eyes return to the young man.

"Now?" the young man asks.

"Right now."

The young man considers. "I feel love," he says finally.

The heavyset man at the center slaps the tabletop. "How merciful is God!" he declares and sits back, satisfied.

Their food arrives, and the men begin to eat. No grace is said. There's little talk as plates are cleared. After the meal a few of the men get up to go, each shaking the hand of the leader on the way out. One older, bald man comes around and sits with the young one who was receiving the attention earlier. They lean forward and huddle close, foreheads inches apart, whispering. When the younger man laughs, the older man squeezes his knee and leaves.

Eventually only the leader and the man on his right remain. I walk over and introduce myself.

"What you witnessed here, Andrew, is our Brotherhood Breakfast. We get together most Saturday mornings, sometimes up to fifty men. And I lead the group for some fellowshipping."

This is Dale. His friend is Jeff. They're members of the Life in Tupelo Pentecostal Church.

"Is this your spot?" I ask, indicating the room, which has nearly filled without my noticing.

"Yes, sir." Dale nods his large head. "We like to spread it around some, but this is usually our gathering place. Preacher often joins us, but he couldn't today. I'm sorry you missed him."

"You seem like a tight-knit group."

"Oh, yes," Jeff says.

"As iron sharpens iron, so a man sharpens the countenance of his friend," Dale recites. "That's from Proverbs 27:17. That's the essence of what we try to do here."

I confess my ignorance of exactly what that means.

"We try and get very intentional, get connected in the right way, and come away better for it."

"The right way?"

"We want to have a conversation, get transparent. It's easy to get together and watch the game, go hunting, play golf—we men tend to deal with the shallow stuff and think we're getting it done. But—and here the ladies have us beat—men don't easily have that conversation, that accountability."

I nod.

"We are all on the struggle bus together."

"The struggle bus?"

"No man is an island, Andrew," Dale quotes John Donne, "entire of itself; every man is a piece of the Continent, a part of the main."

I mention how I was surprised to see such a wide range in ages at the breakfast.

"It's easy to find guys who are like you, but you need diversity, both ethnic and age, to realize we have a lot in common, more than we think. And we live in the day and time of Google and

AI. It's replaced the elder. Google can give you knowledge, but it can't provide wisdom. It's what I'm so proud of with the group. We have friends across generations. And that camaraderie, that friendship is everything."

Then Dale tells me of a friend, a work colleague and fellow Ole Miss football fan, who died by suicide. "That shook me, Andrew. What did I fail to see? That's what's really driven me with the men's group. It's great to go out and shoot the buck of a lifetime and mount it on the wall, but how can I serve? How can I help?

"Women get together, they talk—a real conversation. They notice. We men live behind a facade, and a man needs to be very intentional to take that mask off. That's what we try and do. We all have struggles we are never gonna get over alone, be it pornography or whatever, but we share and take accountability with someone we trust who can receive us without judgment so we can be transformed. We confess our sins to God to be forgiven, we confess our sins to our brother to be healed."

I ask Dale how often he reads the Bible.

"I try to read scripture every day. I fail, like any man does. But it is the words of life."

Dale then invites me to church tomorrow. "We'd be honored to have you."

"I feel like I've just been to church, Dale."

"Well, you've got friends here now." Then Dale places a meaty hand on my shoulder. "The Lord loves you, Andrew, that's a fact."

And with that assurance, I head off to the gun show.

Heading northwest on McCullough Boulevard toward the Tupelo Furniture Market, I find the parking lot nearly full on arrival. Middle-aged men and a surprisingly large number of mature women are coming and going. Only when I walk through the lobby of building two, registering that I didn't have to pay an admission fee, do I notice all the antiques and bric-a-brac spread across hundreds of tables. I approach a stout woman at a folding table in the foyer.

"Um...is this the gun show?" I ask meekly.

"Building five, sweetie," the woman tells me with a smile. "Next parking lot down."

I've never been to a gun show. While I'm not exactly nervous, I am lacking a bit of confidence.

Over at building five the lot is half full, and while there was a buzz surrounding the curios and knickknacks in building two, here things are more muted.

A sign in the lobby of the Tupelo Gun and Knife Show clearly states "No loaded firearms in this building." I pay my $5 and enter.

There's a musty smell to the vast room. Fifty to seventy-five large folding tables have been set up in long rows. Some are covered with knives ("Tactical knives with a bite" one sign boasts), most tables are chock-a-block with firearms—hunting rifles, pistols, tactical weapons, shotguns, assault rifles, and their accompanying accessories, sights, and ammunition.

It's mostly men here, but there are some families, mothers pushing children in strollers. Everyone is white. At a table along one wall, two young fellas, one lean and blond, the other dark-haired and solidly built, are handing out literature about the Libertarian Party. "The Republican Party is like a police state in Mississippi," the dark-haired one tells me. "People don't care, as long as there's an R in front of the name they vote for them. We're just trying to get people to open their eyes."

I ask who the most recent Libertarian candidate for president was. Neither man can tell me. "We're looking to influence things on a local level," the blond says by way of clarification.

At the next table, an AR-15 assault rifle has a price tag hanging from it—$675.

"This one here shoots like an AK-47," the large man with a friendly manner assures me. His name is Ted.

I ask if I can hold it.

"Of course you can." Ted smiles. I pick the gun up. It's lighter than I imagined. "That's a lot of weapon," he assures me.

"I can buy this from you now?" I ask.

"As long as you tell me that you're not a federal criminal."

"I'm not," I assure Ted.

"Then I'm happy to sell it to you."

"I am from out of state, though," I tell Ted.

"Then I just can't sell you a pistol."

A skinny man with a goatee at the next table leans over, and the three of us enter into a spirited discussion of why that is. The law makes no sense to either man, but they assure me good-naturedly they must abide by such stupidity. The two have an easy camaraderie.

"How long you guys been friends?" I ask.

"Too long," Ted says, and they both laugh. "I didn't bring any ammo today"—Ted indicates the assault rifle still in my hands—"but you can get some right over there," and he points to a table two rows away.

I'm not sure what I was expecting, but the atmosphere in the room might best be described as cordially mundane. There's laughing and teasing. Warm greetings are exchanged, as well as considered discussions on firing pins and primers—although there appear to be few sales being made. What I see are normal folks with a common interest, shared sociopolitical beliefs, similar wardrobes. There's a strong sense of solidarity among those present. It all feels pretty workaday.

In one corner, a welcoming guy named Trent is selling handguns. I pick one up.

"Seems like a nice bunch of people," I say, turning the gun in my hand.

"Oh, yeah," Trent says. "It's a close community. We all help each other out." He glances over my shoulder to survey the musty hall. "A lot of solidarity. A lot of friendship in this room."

Oxford, Mississippi

"I feel like I'm somebody who doesn't have a lot of male friends," Tom says. "I don't do a lot of those male-centric activities that men around here do, hunting, or fishing, or golf."

Like any number of men I meet, Tom's wife directs much of his social life. "I'd say Dorothy is my best friend, although I'm not sure she'd say the same about me. We're friends with—or I should say we tend to socialize with—a lot of couples. I have a few friends that, frankly, married people I don't care for and so, consequently, I don't see them much anymore."

It seems there are any number of ways to lose a friend.

I've just met Tom, a thoughtful and professorial-looking architect. We're in a bustling restaurant in Oxford, an hour west of Tupelo along Route 6. A prosperous town and home to the University of Mississippi and the Ole Miss Rebels, Oxford was twice occupied by Union forces during the Civil War, before being burned to the ground. There's a plaque just off the picturesque central square describing the events. As with many similar signs in the South, after reading it, you could be excused for coming away with the impression that the South won the war.

Born in Nashville, Tom's lived in Oxford for more than half a century. "Oxford was the kind of place that when we were young, we couldn't wait to get away from it. Now everybody's coming here. We were a town of six thousand, same size as the university; now we're both twenty thousand."

But numbers aren't the only change. "The square used to be the hub. There was the grocery and hardware, the dry cleaner. Saturday was market day. Everyone came. It was racially diverse, Black and white. Now the square is all boutiques and high-end restaurants like this one. The poor can't afford to come to town, and around here, the poor are the Blacks, so in some ways we've become more segregated, economically segregated."

Besides Ole Miss, Oxford's other claim to fame is the South's greatest twentieth-century writer, William Faulkner.

"I love Faulkner," Tom assures me, "but he's a big forest to walk into."

I confess to not being able to get through any of Faulkner's work since being ground down by *As I Lay Dying* in high school (or, as we called it, *As I Die Reading*).

"I understand," Tom concedes.

"I read a story," I say, "probably apocryphal, but one fine morning, Faulkner went fishing with a friend. Later that afternoon he walked right past the same friend on the street in town without greeting him. Miffed, the man confronted the great writer—'Why would you pass me without saying a word?' Faulkner is said to have replied, 'We just spent the entire morning talking and fishing. What on earth do we have to say to each other?'"

Tom laughs. "My great-uncle was his physician. They were friends, although I'm not sure how many people shared every aspect of Faulkner's life," Tom says diplomatically. "I mean he had his life here writing, his drinking life, and his LA life—and the mistress out there for fifteen years. A complicated man. Have you been to Rowan Oak yet?" Tom asks. "It's just a few blocks away."

And so I go.

While I'm standing on the pillared front porch of Faulkner's antebellum mansion, a soft breeze is blowing through the row of mature eastern red cedars that lead to the home—planted in the common belief that the majestic trees helped to ward off yellow fever. Faulkner named the thirty-three-acre property Rowan Oak for the rowan tree that symbolizes peace and serenity and the oak that represents strength and solitude.

"The place is well named," Rachel Hudson, the assistant curator at Rowan Oak, tells me. "In his life, for the most part, Faulkner was pretty solitary. He didn't rely on friendship. And you don't see the theme of friendship often in Faulkner's work either. Instead, it's race, or family, or class."

I share my fishing story about Faulkner snubbing his friend. Rachel laughs. "That sounds about right. He didn't even want to go collect his Nobel Prize. 'Too far for supper,' he said. His daughter made him go, a year late. He was very much an introvert, not the life of the party. Nor was he universally loved around town."

Oxford stood in for Jefferson, the setting for fifteen of Faulkner's novels. And he was not averse to using its residents as inspiration. "The Compsons, in *The Sound and the Fury*, are well known to have been stand-ins for the Thompsons, a local family," Rachel says. "And not everyone loved the way he represented them, or the South."

A self-professed "yellow dog Democrat," by today's standards Faulkner might be judged unforgivingly for his depiction of Black people. But for his day, he was more progressive than many Southerners, advocating higher education for them in a time when that was far from the prevailing sentiment—contributing portions of his Nobel Prize money to the cause of Black education.

"But he was a hard nut to crack," Rachel concedes.

"Didn't he say, 'I never learned much by talking'?"

"He did."

"Not easy to be friends with that."

"True." Rachel smiles and nods. We stand in silence. The wind picks up. There's something both grand and very human about this place. The grounds have gone a bit to seed. A few outbuildings appear in disrepair, and the bricks of a formal garden that once blossomed rise twisted and pushed up by roots and the years: there to be tripped over. Yet the scraggly yard is welcoming, a peaceful place for a man who didn't like to socialize. It's easy to imagine the writer dragging a small table and typewriter out to work under the trees, as a few of the many photos in the house attest.

The sky, clear blue when I arrived, has begun to cloud over. I admit to Rachel my difficulties in sticking with Faulkner's work.

"He can be tough," Rachel allows, "but the payoff is always worth it."

I promise her I'll give the great writer another try and wander out into the yard. I plant myself in one of the Adirondack chairs scattered by the side of the house, just below Faulkner's bedroom window. I sit for a long, dreamy time. I text Eddie, who I'm on my way to see, for his opinion of Faulkner. Eddie's the most well read of any of my friends.

He responds quickly, *Drank too much! Never could get through a book.*

I put the same question to Matthew. *Hate him. He stole one of my term papers once.* Laughing, I text the same question to Seve. My phone rings. It turns out that Seve knows a fair amount about Faulkner. "Did you know that he went to Canada to join the RAF as a pilot during the First World War?" he informs me. "Because his high school girlfriend dumped him. But the war ended before he could get to battle. So, he went back to Mississippi and became a writer."

"What are you, Mr. Encyclo-fucking-pedia?"

"I literally just ordered his first novel, *A Soldier's Pay*. It should be delivered any day."

"Jesus, Seve, who knew?"

The sky continues to darken. By the time I return to my hotel, the town's tornado siren has sounded, and the sky is filled with ominous, dramatic, low, and shape-shifting gray then black clouds. Tree branches flail in a whirling wind. Traffic lights swing wildly on their wires. No one is on the street. Marble-size hail begins to pelt the ground. The temperature drops—twenty degrees in minutes. Then in less than an hour it's over. Stillness prevails. The next morning—which is bright and calm—I read that six people have been killed in tornadoes where I was just a few days earlier, in Tennessee.

Clarksdale, Mississippi

The word I'm hearing most often to describe Mississippi, from those who live here, is "complicated." Passing through, it's impossible not to feel the weight and legacy of racial oppression.

Leaving the civility of Oxford, I head south-southwest on Route 7. Every few miles buildings announcing themselves as churches appear along the rolling, rural road. None boast a steeple or bell tower. Most just look like houses. There is little sign of human life. The land is washed of color in the hard morning sun. I turn right onto Route 8, past cotton fields left untilled, lifeless gray stalks picked clean save for a few overlooked white tufts clinging to bolls rise twisting and gnarled from pale brown earth. Other fields are fallow. After another half hour, I make a left onto Money Road. The road is ungraded, the poorest I've driven since I left home. Beside me a single telephone wire is strung loosely from pole to pole to pole, dipping and rising again and again in an illusion of movement as I race past. A committee of vultures is feasting on something ahead, in a large, flooded area close beside the road. The pool of water encroaches far out onto the potholed pavement. The scavengers disperse begrudgingly just before my tires spray them. Then, in the rearview mirror, I see the birds land again and resume their meal. The interruption forgotten. The Tallahatchie River winds in and out of view on my right. A railroad track now hugs the road to my left. I slow and pull my car to the side of the road, in front of an abandoned gas station and the ruin of another building.

It's here, inside Bryant's Grocery & Meat Market on the afternoon of August 24, 1955, that the Emmett Till tragedy began. The lynching of the fourteen-year-old Black boy from Chicago by two white men would prove a defining spark in igniting the civil rights movement.

There's no one around. The field across the street, beyond the railroad track, is plowed under and lifeless. The wind blows under a cold sun.

It's just the decaying shell of the grocery where the young Till reportedly whistled at a white woman. The roof and windows are long gone, the front porch has collapsed, its brick walls crumbling and kept up principally by tangled vines that encase and strangle the structure. There's nothing, other than a small nearby plaque, to suggest what was set in motion here. Nothing has been preserved.

Heading north on US 49, I make a right onto the optimistically named Swan Lake Road. The crudely patched macadam crosses over the railroad tracks, then over the Tallahatchie and onto River Road—loose yellow stones over two lonely miles, past long-abandoned fields.

A prominent steamboat anchorage in 1840, Graball Landing is now nothing but a small, desolate clearing in the trees, exposing a sweeping bend and the lazy flow of the Tallahatchie. Birds sing, a bright red cardinal lands on a bare tree limb above the brown water. It's here where Till's bloated, nearly unrecognizable body, still wrapped in barbed wire, was said to have been pulled from the river. In 2004, a plaque was erected commemorating the site. The sign, just as Till had been, was thrown in the river. A second sign was put up and soon shot full of holes. As was a third. The plaque that stands now is bulletproof.

Eleven miles up the road in tiny Sumner (population 260), an outsize Richardsonian Romanesque courthouse dominates the slip of a town. Up a flight of creaking wooden stairs is the courtroom that housed the Till murder trial. A recent renovation has ensured it looks much as it did in 1955. There is no reference to the events that took place here. The room where twelve white jurors hastily freed Till's murderers is empty. My steps echo.

The events of those horrific days surrounding Till's lynching have been revisited and reevaluated over the years, the evidence scoured over and reexamined, then examined again. Best-selling books have been written about the tragedy, interviews recorded, films and documentaries have been made. I can offer no insight, nor have I any authority to do so—yet every traveler discovers the already explored world for themselves.

On the sidewalk in the bright sun in front of a deserted shop directly across the street from the courthouse, a dead sparrow is lying on the pavement—it probably flew into the plate-glass window boarded up from the inside. One wing is splayed unnaturally. The bird's twiglike talons are curling at their tips. I ease it off the pavement into the nearby long grass.

Just a half hour up Route 49 from Sumner, you could be excused for dismissing ravaged Clarksdale with a cursory glance—that would be a mistake. John Lee Hooker was born here. So was Sam Cooke. So was Ike Turner, who as a boy worked as an elevator operator at the Alcazar Hotel on Third Street. Bessie Smith died here. Muddy Waters grew up just down the road at Stovall Plantation. And at the crossroads on the edge of town, Robert Johnson was said to have sold his soul to the devil so he could play the blues like no other. Perhaps no one place can be said to be the birthplace of the blues, but Clarksdale, Mississippi, can lay a pretty fair claim.

As is the case with so much of Mississippi, first appearances are deceiving. There's a muffled current running through town that its boarded-up storefronts and taped-over windows mask. A good many of those shuttered-looking places, once you push open the door, are pulsing—or at least have a pulse.

Over in the lobby of the Travelers Hotel—which once housed a brothel—I encounter two men who grew up in Clarksdale and recall better days.

"We came along at a time when this town was ripe for people, white people, to thrive," Chuck Rutledge tells me. "The railroad track divide was very real, but for us it was a true Mayberry type existence." Chuck, who runs this hotel with his wife, Ann, is fair-haired and still boyish. He grew up here in the 1970s with his friend Dan Crumpton, a farmer.

"We never locked our door, rode our bikes everywhere. Keys were left in the car," Dan says, wearing a baseball cap and sporting a trim beard. His hard blue eyes soften the longer we talk. "It was an idyllic childhood."

Dan is extroverted and direct. Chuck is introverted, considered. Both left town to go to college, Dan to Ole Miss and Chuck to New Orleans. Both stayed away for years. Both eventually moved back.

They've been the closest of friends their entire lives.

"Every Friday night, I was over at his house, or he was at mine," Chuck says.

"His mother used to make these amazing doughnuts." Dan laughs. "She'd slice them open, put butter on 'em, and toast them."

Both men almost swoon at the memory.

"That, with a glass of milk and watching cartoons." Chuck shakes his head. "It didn't get better."

"The thing about our relationship," Dan says, "is our fathers were childhood friends. They grew up together, hunted together, and were dear friends all their lives till Chuck's dad died."

"Tell him about the hogs," Chuck prompts his friend to share a famous family story involving their fathers, as boys, being chased by wild hogs on an island while skinny-dipping in the Mississippi and losing their clothes. "Real Huck Finn, Mark Twain stuff." Chuck shakes his head.

"And our grandfathers—his grandfather Otis and my grandfather Big Dan—were best friends. That's three generations." Dan holds up three fingers to prove the point.

Chuck nods. "We saw our fathers being best friends their whole lives. It's learned behavior. That legacy, we appreciate it carries some of the weight, and we can count on that, but it only takes you so far. For example, I had surgery several years ago in New Orleans and I wake up and first thing I see is Dan staring down at me. He didn't live in New Orleans, but he was there."

Not to be outdone, Dan shows me a long scar on his neck. "See that? I had a lump here. Of course I ignored it. Everyone said to go to the doctor. I didn't listen. Chuck insisted. He made the appointment, made me go. Long story short, it was a malignant melanoma in my lymph nodes." Dan points to his friend. "I wouldn't have listened to anyone else. He saved my life."

"So, there's that." Chuck smiles.

"Look, we're pretty different individuals," Dan goes on. "Politically we're other ends of the spectrum. Socially, I'm outgoing. Chuck keeps to himself. Doesn't matter. Doesn't come into play. Our friendship is just a given. It was established from day one. We never even questioned it. I think this is the first time we've ever even talked about it."

Chuck nods. "Even when we haven't seen each other, lived in different places, didn't talk much, doesn't matter."

I look over the top of my tea. "Aristotle said, 'Separation doesn't destroy friendship absolutely, though it prevents its active exercise.'"

"Well"—Dan pushes back his cap—"Aristotle didn't grow up on the Mississippi Delta. I can tell you that for sure."

Chuck smiles at his friend. "We're friends. And we know that."

As was the case with Lew and Bobby back in Ohio, I comprehend what these two are telling me and understand it on an intellectual level, but despite how close I may be with my friends, I can only envy the solidity such a lifelong friendship might offer.

"It's special," Dan says, "and it's rare and it's generational. And the older I get the more I appreciate it."

"I'd guess that appreciation compounds its rewards."

"That's very true, Andrew." Dan nods slowly. "It does."

"So, what the hell happened to town?" I ask.

Chuck sighs. "I call it a perfect storm of big-box retail and manufacturing moving out of the country. When you start losing the mom and pops"—he shrugs—"they can't compete with Walmart. All of a sudden there's a lack of opportunity and people with economic mobility leave, to Oxford or Memphis, and you're left with landowners and poor people. The divide grows. That's how you go from twenty-five thousand to fifteen like we have now."

"These streets were packed growing up. That building right there." Dan points across the street to a five-story abandoned office building. "Lawyers, accountants, dentists. I remember having my teeth drilled and looking out onto this parking lot—they had a carnival going on, with that tilt-a-whirl thing going around."

"This was the same dentist that used to give us a ball of mercury to play with to distract us," Chuck remembers. "It would split into perfect little balls when you dropped it on the tray. Lot of fun."

"Yeah." Dan laughs. "It was poison."

The one thing that is helping to bring Clarksdale back from the brink is the blues. Over on Delta Avenue, Roger Stolle, the owner of Cat Head Delta Blues & Folk Art, an emporium of all things blues, has been helping to lead that charge, trying "to promote the blues from within" for the past twenty years. He's quick to admit the challenges they face. "There's no way to come into Clarksdale and have it present well. I mean, a place that looks this tired…"

"Tired?" I say. "The entire town looks like it could be condemned."

"But the music brings people out and brings them together," Roger goes on. "We're nearly eighty percent Black, less than twenty percent white, but there's a global friendship through the blues. It's a unifier. We may be on the other side of the walls politically, culturally, economically, but the blues brings us together. The blues is survival music. We can all identify and relate to that. Around here you got church or the blues. Church is in direct competition with the juke joint. There's only so much money. It's going one of two places. That's why the church labeled the blues the devil's music.

"And there's the live element of both. You put people in a space where they can experience that connection. In church it's from the pulpit. The juke joint is a house party thrown by a guy who doesn't want you in his house."

One such juke joint sits on the edge of town by the banks for the Sunflower River. It's a broke-down ruin of a place called Red's Lounge. Blues man Lucious Spiller is on the bill tonight. Red is at home, ailing, so I give my ten-dollar cover charge to Ellis, a tall man who doesn't move so much as glide under a tall cowboy hat. For another dollar Ellis slides me a warm can of Coke eased from the portable red cooler behind the bar. There's no stage here, just an open floor covered by an expanse of carpet that fell off the back of the truck delivering new rugs to a riverside casino in Vicksburg. Along one wall is the bar and a row of stools. Opposite the bar is a set of drums. The musicians—depending on how many show up—cluster around the drums to play. In the back are a few mismatched tables. I take a seat in a row of chairs by the door. A heap of discarded boxes and assorted trash is crowded behind me and piled high in the corner. The place feels like someone's living room who has lived far too long without seeing the light of day and has no access to a dumpster. The bathroom is a fright. It's perhaps the most delicious venue for music I've ever encountered.

Lucious arrives and begins messing with his guitar. He, Ellis, and I are the only ones in the place. Sufficiently warmed up, Lucious wanders over. He is still wearing his wool hat and scarf, which he will wear the entire evening. Lucious had a stroke several years ago and had to learn to play all over again. "It's frustrating," the bluesman confesses. "I tell my fingers what to do, but they don't always listen anymore."

Originally from St. Louis, Lucious came to Clarksdale, like so many, to play the blues. He looks exhausted, used by life, but he's amiable with an easy smile.

"It's been slow lately," he says, looking around at the empty club, "but if it's just you, I love to play, and I'll give you what I got."

Eventually a drummer, harmonica player, bassist, and guitar player wander in. A mix of white and Black men. A couple from Cincinnati whom I met earlier on the street come in and settle at a table. Lucious is true to his word. For ninety minutes the five musicians give it up for the three of us in attendance. I've been to shows in clubs, arenas, and stadiums filled with 80,000 people, and rarely experienced a more thrilling evening of music.

After, on the street I fall into conversation with the lead guitarist, Grayson, with whom Lucious seemed to be the most in sync, trading licks and handing off one to the other with effortless musicality. The two men couldn't seem more different. Lucious is a Black man of indeterminate age, who moves under the weight of the world. Grayson is a pale-skinned, blond and blue-eyed bright spirit from Idaho. He came to Clarksdale four years ago to play the blues.

"Me and Lucious play about once a week. We don't talk much, but I understand a good deal about him, and him me. I'm probably closer to him than just about anybody in town. He's my closest friend. And it's through the music."

The next morning I'm on the street early. Town is deserted. It feels postapocalyptic. Last night's music is still in my head.

A large, black and brown mixed-breed dog silently waddles up behind me, her mammaries swinging heavy and full of milk. She falls in with me and we walk, turn for turn, through town. We come upon no one, and I appreciate her company. Arriving at Our

Grandma's House of Pancakes, the canine sits, looking in at me as the sun streaks through a large plate-glass window in dire need of Windex. I'm the only customer. The walls are a stained yellow and covered in torn and faded photos of people I don't know. The vinyl tablecloth is sticky. The pancakes are light and delicious. Two local women come in to pick up a take-out order. We make idle, satisfying, chitchat. Neither of the women know the dog.

I wrap one of my pancakes in a paper napkin. Outside, the dog looks up with watery eyes, then swallows the pancake in two bites. I touch her for the first time, patting her head. Friends without words. She hoists herself to her feet and finally lumbers off, mammaries swinging low and rhythmic. I watch until she turns the corner.

Highway 1 South bisects tilled fields, brown and rowed earth stretching for miles. A lack of money exposes a place, and the land along the Delta feels exciting in its elemental unadornment. An hour south, on the banks of the Mississippi River, is another iconic stop along the blues trail, Rosedale. Eric Clapton famously sang of the town in the Cream classic "Crossroads." (Like Clarksdale and a few other towns, Rosedale claims to be the actual crossroads where Robert Johnson made his deal with the devil.) Inspiring Clapton decades earlier, Johnson himself immortalized Rosedale in his song "Traveling Riverside Blues," suggesting to his baby that she "squeeze my lemon till the juice run down my leg."

There isn't a lot flowing these days in Rosedale. More than half the population of nearly two thousand lives below the poverty level, ranking it among the poorest towns in the poorest state in the country.[1] Side streets of humble dignity are interspersed among those with shotgun shacks and overgrown lawns. Rusted cars sit on cinder blocks. On the corner of Main and Brown is a small white house—the White Front Café–Joe's Hot Tamale Place.

"Hot tamales and they're red hot, yes she's got 'em for sale" sang Johnson in another of his classic, innuendo-filled blues numbers. Barbara, the woman behind the counter, may not be exactly who Johnson was singing about, but she's got an easy, if exhausted, charm. The tamales are prepared on a simple kitchen stove, a nearby sign warns of "Absolutely No Credit." It's take-out only these days, but when I gesture toward the few tables with red-and-white checkerboard vinyl covers, Barbara shrugs and busies herself at the stove. I busy myself eating. The silence of our shared company fills the room with something the silence of solitude can't. For the moment at least, friends without words.

Natchitoches, Louisiana

I wake to an email from my friend Don, who was in Japan when I first reached out to him while sitting at the kitchen table back in New York.

Hey A!!! Just back from two amazing months in Japan! How are you? Where are you??

My friend's ebullient nature comes through even in an email. Few people can communicate with punctuation the way Don can.

In Mississippi. Ever been? I type quickly and press send.

Continuing down Highway 1 on the western edge of Mississippi, my intent is to cross the Big Muddy, bisect Louisiana, cross into Texas, and meet up with my friend Eddie in Cleburne, south of Dallas, in a few days' time.

In the Civil War town of Vicksburg, I've no interest in visiting the famous battleground commemorating the siege in which the Union Army cleaved the South in half, cementing General Ulysses S. Grant's reputation. Nor do the riverfront casinos hold any allure.

Crossing the river here would commit me to Interstate 80 for the entire width of Louisiana. Since I'm doing everything I can on this trip to avoid those four/six/eight-lane thoroughfares of stress, I continue south on local Highway 61 down through the Delta. But I'm tired of driving. My back aches. I'm hungry. My impulsive road trip seems to have suddenly caught up to me.

In Natchez I walk the promenade for a good look at the mighty Mississippi. The great river is low, its high mudbanks exposed and scarred. The brown water appears almost stagnant—until I notice a large floating tree branch moving at a deceptive pace downstream.

I'd like to feel that on this trip, despite its improvisational quality, I'm moving with similarly deceptive certainty toward something of value. Like the branch buoyed by the river, I'm being supported and propelled by the vast, complex, and contradictory country I've been inching through, over thousands of unanticipated miles, meeting men along the way willing to offer up their insights and experiences, illuminating and clarifying the value and import of friendship. But right now, the road is a grind. I feel untethered, alone. Solitude is often a condition I relish. Today, it all just feels empty.

Louisiana greets me in the way I'm greeted by much of the South—Sonic Drive-In, Dollar General, fallow fields, poverty. I'm just driving. West along Highway 84, I stop for pleasant service and bad barbecue at the Brisket House in lifeless Jena. I'm not giving Louisiana much of a chance. God save the traveler who has been abandoned by curiosity.

A few hours west, I pull into the eighteenth-century town of Natchitoches. With wrought iron balconies lining the Cane River, its charms are obvious. I try to rally.

Sometimes doors swing wide to welcome a wanderer as if preordained, yet at other times joyless trudging spawns dissatisfaction that feels like a foregone conclusion.

Everywhere I try to get a room is full.

"Fuck," I curse to my otherwise empty car. I've parked on the side of the road to scroll my phone, looking for a place to hang my head as the sky loses light. I find a bed-and-breakfast. Apparently the 1989 movie *Steel Magnolias* starring Julia Roberts was filmed in town and a scene or two was shot at this B&B. The we're-all-friends-who-just-haven't-met-yet sensibility common to many bed-and-breakfasts is one I try to avoid, but I'm in no mood for the potluck of the roadside motel, the likes of which I've been perfectly content with often enough on this trip. After a weary afternoon, I'm looking for a softer landing tonight.

When I call, I'm relieved to be offered the last available room, the renovated attic. I leap at it. Only then do I ask the price. It's triple what I have paid anywhere since leaving home. "Fine," I grumble and ask for directions.

The house is walking distance from the postcard-ready town center and along the river. It's a handsome brick home dating back to the mid-nineteenth century with a welcoming porch shaded by out-of-season wisteria.

There's no one there to receive me but I've been given a door code. It's wrong. When I call the same number I used to book the room ten minutes earlier there is no answer. I sit on the back stoop to wait. Eventually another guest returns, and only after considering the bag at my feet and my expression, allows me access. Walking in, I'm confronted by Dolly Parton and Sally Field arguing with Shirley MacLaine on a large television playing *Steel Magnolias* on a loop. I climb the stairs.

Up a lovely wide and wooden staircase, the doors to three bedrooms are propped open, revealing spaces any grandmother would be proud to sleep in, with four-poster beds, candlesticks, and quilts. I relax and keep climbing. Two of the doors on the next floor are closed, and the third room appears similar to those below—it even has a cozy looking window seat. I keep climbing.

The attic door is propped open. My room does not look like the others. It looks like a storage space with a sagging bed shoved against the wall. The faux-leather couch in the corner is stained. The toilet runs, no matter how much I jiggle the handle. The bathroom light is burnt out. There is no soap in the plastic shower stall. I feel like I'm Rochester's first wife in *Jane Eyre*, sequestered in the attic.

I pull out my phone to see if perhaps I can switch to one of the other more welcoming and as yet unoccupied rooms I passed on my climb. There's no service, and I decide to go down for a better signal. The door swings closed behind me. Once in the hall I realize how stuffy the room was and reach back to prop it open. But the door is now locked. I have no key.

I finally make contact with someone on the phone and am informed that all the other rooms are fully spoken for. I mention my locked door and am met with silence.

"Hello?" I say.

"Um, the key wasn't in the door?" the voice asks tentatively.

"No."

"Hmm, that one locks automatically."

"I discovered that."

I'm instructed to go into a storage room by the kitchen. There I find a large rack of keys, some labeled, many not.

"Is there anyone who can come help me?"

"Well, I'm making dinner here at home, but the extra key is there. Just look around. It's there on that rack."

I spend the next thirty minutes going up and down the stairs until I find a loose and unlabeled key that fits.

One of the great benefits of travel is that it often aligns us with who we would like to be, relieved of daily irritants or familiar routine. Consequently, less-than-ideal or even miserable circumstances can be viewed through the prism of a unique experience, a one-time pleasure, or as Seve likes to remind me, experienced "for the story we can tell." And that's been my attitude at every stop, however modest or peculiar, but this obvious money grab—coupled with my road fatigue—has defeated my traveler's optimism.

On bustling Front Street, below the wrought iron balconies and hanging lights reflecting off the river, people parade with cocktails in to-go cups. Others dip small spoons into scoops of ice cream. I slip into a restaurant but can't decide and walk out only to return five minutes later and my spot is gone. Eventually I find a corner seat at the bar of a middling restaurant and eat overcooked fish. Beside me at the bar is a trim man. He wears large clear-framed glasses over pale blue eyes, is cleanshaven with skin drawn tight over an angular face. He's in Natchitoches with his wife, to visit her sister. When he inquires what I'm doing in town, I tell him I'm passing through, and why.

"Huh," he grunts. "That sounds like a nice thing to do."

"It is. Although today hasn't been the greatest day of my life."

"Those days are difficult to come by." His manner is gruff, irritated, but it seems that's just his habitual way and has nothing to do with anything passing between us. Regardless, it's difficult to relax under such a presence—which I get the feeling is exactly the way that this man likes it.

I'm conscious we haven't exchanged names.

He sips his beer and is silent. Then he surprises me.

"I don't think I could do what you're doing," he says.

"Why's that?"

"Well." He catches the bartender's eye and lifts his empty glass, ordering another beer. "I had a good friend. We had a falling-out several years back."

"Sorry to hear that."

"Yeah."

We both look up at the hockey game playing on the television behind the bar. Back and forth, up and down the ice they race. When he's finished most of his next beer, and still staring at the TV, he says, "Maybe I'll give him a call."

I glance over. "Probably couldn't hurt at this point." Then I instantly regret my comment. "I mean…" I stumble. "It's been good to see my friends, so…maybe…"

He glares at me.

The next morning, I descend the stairs early to the sound of someone setting a modest buffet in the kitchen—the first person who works at the B&B that I've encountered face-to-face. I place my key on the counter and mutter, "Thank you."

"Did you enjoy your stay?" the lively woman in floral dress and frilled apron wants to know.

I hesitate. "Are you asking?" I say, knowing there is no point. This woman is a hired hand. None of it is her fault.

"Why, yes. Was something wrong?" She couldn't be sweeter.

So I tell her—from being locked out, twice, to the bad bed and broken bath to the exorbitant price. This place provided no welcome, offered no hospitality. "No one bothered to show up when they were needed."

The woman visibly shudders. I knew I shouldn't have started. She doesn't deserve any of this, and she seems genuinely horrified I did not have a fabulous stay. "Well, I will most certainly pass this along, and I'm sure you will be offered some kind of a refund."

"It's not necessary," I tell her. "I'm sorry I brought you into it."

"Between us, darlin'"—the woman lowers her voice—"I think sometimes they think since they were in a movie that they're something a little bit special."

"Well, I was in a movie and I still ended up sleeping in Mr. Rochester's attic."

"Huh?"

"Don't mind me." I turn to go. "Have a good day."

"Are you sure you don't want to take a biscuit with you?"

I just want out. I throw my bag in the car and pick up El Camino Real headed west.

Alto, Texas

The Greek philosopher Epicurus was correct when he said, "It is not so much our friends' help that helps us as the confident knowledge that they will help us." I know this because as I come off the causeway over the Toledo Bend reservoir separating Louisiana and Texas, I feel my shoulders relax.

I'd gotten used to the shadow of constant anxiety at the warning on my dash reading "Maintenance—Tire," as it has since I was with Matthew in Kentucky. Add to that at some point near the Mississippi River it began alternating with a more ominous warning announcing "Maintenance—Other." But suddenly I don't care anymore. I'm in Texas now, home of my oldest friend, Eddie. And even though I am still hundreds of miles and hours of driving away, I know he'll come get me if need be.

I met Eddie in high school. He was my English teacher for a semester during the fall of my senior year. Having graduated from Columbia University just the year before, Eddie was seven years older than me—and a world more worldly. While other teachers at school wore penny loafers and button-down shirts, Eddie cruised around in retro 1950s suits and skinny ties. He rode a motorcycle and lived in Greenwich Village—an exotic and distant planet from my nearby New Jersey suburb. I admired him hugely, but mostly from a distance.

Then, in an audacious and out-of-character move, when I came to New York City the following autumn to attend NYU, I pressed the buzzer on the door of his five-story walk-up on Bank Street. Eddie's head popped out of a top-floor window. I shouted up a nervous greeting, and he withdrew. Sure that I had overstepped my bounds, I began to walk away only to hear my name. I look up. Eddie had reappeared out the window and was holding something in his hand. "Catch," he shouted and tossed down a key wrapped in a dish towel. I turned the lock, climbed the five flights, and presented myself for friendship.

Eddie's acceptance of me was instantaneous and complete. And still surprises me.

Eddie did more to influence who I would become than anyone, and my relationship with him changed my place in the world forever. Suddenly, because of Eddie, a chasm had been crossed. His was my first adult friendship. Not only New Jersey, but the childhood I had been aching to discard was suddenly behind me. My life had begun at last, and I felt that I couldn't have had a better guide.

Soon I was dressing in the same baggy clothes procured from the secondhand shops along Eighth Street, going to the revival house movie theaters that would become my obsession, and walking around with folded-up newspapers in my back pocket—the *Times* in the morning and the *Daily News* in the afternoon. (I would later adopt this look for my role in the movie *St. Elmo's Fire* and base my portrayal of my character in *Weekend at Bernie's* on Eddie—if Eddie had been a complete idiot.) We shot pool at Julian's Billiard Hall on Fourteenth Street with the old men and petty crooks. We drank McSorley's dark ale at the bucket-of-blood bar on his corner. We raced around on his dilapidated motorcycle. I even started putting mustard on my cheeseburgers because Eddie did.

We talked and laughed. He listened to me; he was interested. He valued my opinions. He respected who I inherently was—I had never experienced that. For a scared kid new to the city who felt so separate from the others at college, his surprising friendship was an unlikely lifeline. And I can't recall the last time I've seen him.

But first I have to cross east Texas. I'd have known I was in the Lone Star State even without seeing the sign that reads "Drive Friendly, the Texas Way." As I crossed the border the speed limit on rolling, winding, pine-lined, two-lane Route 21 suddenly increased to seventy miles per hour, and I'm now being passed by Ford F-150 pickup trucks as if standing still.

Despite my eagerness to see my friend, the traveling blues I acquired in Louisiana still cling to me. This isn't helped when I receive an email from last night's bed-and-breakfast. Management heard that certain aspects of my stay were "less than perfect" and have offered me a ten percent discount on my next visit. I delete the message.

Farther west, on the street in tiny Alto, Texas, I stop to stretch my legs and pop into Miss Mollie's Diner, with a large sign out front boasting "Service as sweet as the tea." Both things prove to be true, and while that makes the experience pleasant, it makes the tea undrinkable for this Yankee. Once outside, I see a man with a long and full white beard wearing a mesh baseball cap and plaid shirt. His large belt buckle is nearly obscured beneath his protruding belly. As I approach, he takes a seat on a bench out front of the Cherokee County Republican Party headquarters. The man and I nod gravely to each other. Just then an eighteen-wheeler pulling an oversize flatbed carrying some kind of ventilation fan larger than I thought possible is struggling to make a sharp turn. All surrounding activity stops. Cars in every direction reverse to make room. When the truck has navigated the turn and moved on, the man with the long beard and I meet eyes again. This time he raises his eyebrows, purses his lips and nods his head, impressed.

I return the gesture.

Something in this particular interaction penetrates me and, in an instant, the steepening slide of sagging spirits I've been experiencing since crossing the Mississippi is reversed.

"I'm Andrew," I say before I know I'm doing it and stick out my hand, as if reaching for the lifeline this man has thrown me.

"Ted," the man with the long beard says, grabbing my hand. "Pleasure to meet you, Andrew."

"Likewise, Ted."

We each nod again. This is the entirety of our relationship. Heading back to my car, I conclude that I like this charmless crossroads of a town quite a lot.

Buckling in, I check my email. Don—who has never responded to an email with the neurotic speed of someone like, say, me—has returned my email from a few days earlier.

Mississippi??!! WOW! Never been, always wanted to go. What are you doing there??

I laugh, my empty car suddenly filled with good feeling. I type, *In Texas now*, and hit send.

Up the road an hour in hardscrabble Palestine, I treat myself to lunch in the once grand Redlands Hotel. I'm seated beside a long table of sixteen middle-aged women dressed for success. Their gathering is filled with laughter and borders on raucous.

"What's the occasion?" I ask as I stand to pay my bill.

"It's Wednesday," drawls a diminutive woman in a lime-green pantsuit with a large gold pendant. Her hair, expertly sculpted and frozen high in place, would make Margaret Thatcher envious.

"Every Wednesday?" I ask.

"Every Wednesday, sweetie," says a tall blonde in full pancake makeup with impressive shoulder pads and ropes of gold around her neck.

Laughter erupts at the far end of the table. "Good to have friends," I say.

"It sure is, darlin'," another blonde halfway down the table calls out, lifting her white wine. The ladies toast themselves, laughing.

Why are women just so much better at this?

I charge along Route 287, and the land and sky yawn open near Corsicana. By the time I've gotten to Waxahachie it looks like Texas—flat and unspeakably vast.

I'm surrounded now by power lines and factories and telephone wires. Flatbed trucks haul long steel rods. Cement mixers turn. Speed traps lurk. I encounter my first bout with traffic since Nashville.

On the outskirts of Cleburne, a town of thirty thousand named for a Confederate general, cattle graze in a field under electrical wires across the road from J&J Donuts and an RV sales lot. Beside the railyard in the parking lot of The Tire Store, a Texas state trooper's SUV sits with its lights flashing, while an officer leans on the door of a nearby white pickup, talking to the several Latino men crammed into the cabin.

On the corner of North Anglin and East Chambers Streets, across from the barbershop, down the block from the Rugged

Man boutique, and around the corner from the Jeans, Jewels, and Jesus secondhand shop, I turn into the parking lot behind an old and venerable building plainly under construction and park beside a full dumpster. The gray metal door is shoved open.

Eddie comes out, squinting against the late-afternoon light like he's emerging from one of the after-hours clubs we used to frequent downtown back in the day. He's wearing purple high-top Converse sneakers and dressed in customary cutoff army fatigues and torn T-shirt. His thinning hair is pulled back in a long ponytail.

"My brother!" he calls out, and we embrace.

I follow my friend into a large, windowed storefront under construction. Twenty-five years ago, after leaving New York for several years of wandering—first to teach English in Thailand, later working at a sports book in Las Vegas—Eddie returned home to Dallas and began buying and renovating old buildings.

He introduces me to a few of the men he's working with, and we head to his apartment one flight up. He's just finished renovating a dozen living spaces, busting through some walls, stripping back the floors, exposing the old tin ceiling. He moved into one himself a week earlier, boxes are still everywhere. Eddie offers me a root beer and one of the only two chairs in the place, a wooden rocker. He sits in a straight-back chair and puts his feet up on a milk carton, and wants to hear about my trip, where I've been, how Seve really is.

"Oh, crap," Eddie responds when I describe our last meeting, and the degree of pain I saw Seve in. "I didn't think I was getting the full story when I talked to him."

This leads us directly into the topic of friendship.

"When you start to pull punches it starts the deterioration of the relationship," Eddie says, summing up what goes wrong with pretty much every relationship.

And then I'm confessing how I've become "bad" at friendship.

"What does that mean?"

"I suppose it started after my divorce."

"From Carol? That was twenty years ago."

"I guess I withdrew."

"What for?"

"I don't know, I felt like some people took sides."

Eddie scrunches up his face in an I'm-not-really-buying-that face.

I shrug. "I guess I felt guilty, ashamed."

"But are friends not the family we get to choose?"

"Well, that's the saying, right? I guess because I never felt close or connected to my family growing up, I never liked that line."

"But you're close to your mom."

I go into some of the recent details of my mother's deteriorating health and mental condition. Eddie shakes his head. He has long firsthand experience with the ravages and cruelty of mental decline. Both his father and sister suffered for years with dementia. "I wouldn't wish it on my worst enemy," Eddie says. "My sister, she had early onset and was very, very clear, she did not want to end up in a home the way she did for so long. The shit that was happening to her…"

"I don't know what your sister's feelings were," I say, "and a lot of people say that, but in the end, they cling to life. I see my mother, her quality of life is awful, she doesn't understand what the hell is going on, but I see her very literally fighting for her life every single day. We just have to honor that instinct."

Eddie is quiet, then, "Yeah."

My rocking chair squeaks with each forward and back and we sip root beer. It's a fairly intense conversation for two guys who have not seen each other in years to launch in on.

"I think the last great lesson I can give my kids is how to die," Eddie says matter-of-factly.

He asks what Rowan, my youngest, is into these days, and Willow, my daughter. And Sam. We talk about his oldest, Bradley, now an EMT, who I knew a little as a child. And Jessie Rey, at college now.

"I loved being a dad to young kids," Eddie says with gusto. "It really surprised me how much I loved it. I was all in. Speaking of which"—Eddie glances around for his phone—"those kids both just ghosted the fuck out of me." He laughs—it's a cackling kind of adolescent giggle.

Eddie went through hell in an ugly divorce decades ago, traveling to San Francisco from Dallas every two weeks for several troubled years until he was granted full custody. I joined him on a few of those weekend trips, hunkering down at a roadside motel while Eddie's awkward visits were initially monitored. I learned a lot about love and humility and showing up and consistency, watching my friend on those grueling weekends.

We get up and he starts to show me how he's renovated the place, and Eddie returns to the topic of kids. "I mess with the idea of foster care, or mentoring," he says. "But then I think I'm just too selfish."

"You'd love it," I say. "And you'd be great at it."

He equivocates. "Nah, it scares me how much I like being alone."

"Tell me about it. But you're a total extrovert."

Eddie scrunches his face again. "I'd say I'm an introvert with decent extrovert qualities. I happen to be very interested in people's stories. But ultimately, I think I have very little faith in people."

"That's just your defensiveness talking. Not wanting to get hurt."

"Maybe. But I do know that most people want to talk, and few people want to listen. I want every nook and cranny."

To prove his point, that night we're at dinner across the street at a small coffee shop by day that in the evenings becomes Jimmy's Steak House, where Eddie engages our waitress. Violetta, tall and rail thin, grew up in town. ("All we had back then was the roller rink.") She fled as a young woman only to return fifteen years ago to be with her ailing father. She teaches dance a few days a week at the Wonderland Dance Academy around the corner. Violetta was also married once.

"He had no friends. No one." She shakes her head and hum/groans for emphasis. "Mmmm-mm. He was smothering me. I was like, 'Step back. I don't know much about being a man. You go find someone. Go have your time, 'cause I need mine.'"

"You think your partner should be your best friend?" Eddie asks.

"I don't know about that." Violetta shakes her head. "Y'all are so shut down," and she makes a gesture with her hand from high to low, as if behind a wall. "I don't know what this whole taboo thing with emotions is about between you guys."

"Well," Eddie says, "the whole gay thing."

"That's just stupid," Violetta snaps, thrusting her hip out hard. "I tell you this for nothing. We were both broken. Thought I could fix him. Humph," she scoffs. "Well, I'm not broke no more."

Only a fool would challenge Violetta standing over us, staring down, hands on hips.

"Women are just so far out ahead of men," Eddie says, and mentions a town council in Minnesota that is all women. "I think maybe I ought to move there."

"Yeah," Violetta says. "Me too."

Cleburne, Texas

The following morning, crossing over Main Street behind a filthy white pickup, Eddie is lamenting the state of things in his home state, and the hard political swing Texas has taken to the right. "You got a lot of good folks here. They don't want their daughter delivering a rapist's baby—they just got conned into something."

We enter the R&K Café II. "I don't know where number one is," Eddie preempts my question.

It's a large, open, and square room with well-spaced wooden tables and chairs. (As a New Yorker, I'm always surprised to see how much room tables are given out in the rest of America.) A wagon wheel hangs from one wall. Paintings of cowboys roping steer hang from another. The ceiling fans are idle. A sign behind the register reads "Happy Trails," and one over the bathroom says "Hold Your Horses." The place is full and boisterous. There are men with large bellies and beards under mesh caps, some families with small children. There are a lot of hoodies and Carhartt jackets. Waitresses hurry by with large plates of pancakes as well as biscuits and gravy crawling up their arms.

Like he did with so many things, Eddie first introduced me to the joys of breakfast in a diner when I was a young and impressionable college freshman and mimicking his every move. Around the corner from his apartment in Greenwich Village, there was, and still is, the greasiest of greasy spoons in the city. Nothing about the place has changed since I first walked into it in

1980—my wife, who is game for most experiences, refuses to eat there. Yet it has always felt to me like a haven, like home. It must be why I love and seek out diners to this day. I mention all this to Eddie.

"Well, little brother, we are connected." We haven't reminisced since my arrival, but now we laugh about past exploits, road trips, and drunken nights.

Then I press Eddie to take me a half hour north into Dallas to the Sixth Floor Museum at Dealey Plaza, from where Lee Harvey Oswald is said to have shot President Kennedy. He grumbles but acquiesces.

It's a deceptively comprehensive experience, detailing both the Warren Commission report that stands as history's official record and the various conspiracy theories that have long endured. After standing in the exact spot from where Oswald was said to have shot Kennedy, Eddie concludes it could not have gone down the way the Warren Commission said.

"That was absolutely fascinating," Eddie—who had never been to the museum and had no interest in going—confesses as we drive back toward Cleburne into a glaring afternoon sun.

"See, dude," I gloat. "So, you know what we get to do next?"

"Oh, no." He cackles like a boisterous adolescent. "Be afraid, be very afraid. What?"

The Fort Worth Stock Show and Rodeo is currently on at Dickies Arena.

"No. Absolutely not. No fucking way," he says.

"Have you ever been?"

"Never."

"You're a Texan and you've never been to the rodeo?"

"You ever been to the Statue of Liberty?"

"Never."

"Exactly."

Eddie drives. The glare of the sun off the eight-lane highway is almost blinding. "Okay," he says finally, "if you're going to the rodeo you need to get some cowboy boots first."

"Now you're talking."

"Pointed toe or round?" Eddie quizzes.

"Pointed," I reply.

"Correct."

Only then does Eddie take the exit, and the blinding sun falls harmless over our shoulder. He guides me through the Near Southside of Fort Worth, shows me a few of the earlier properties he renovated, and then over to Justin's Outlet on Vickery Boulevard.

Boots. Floor to ceiling. Pointed toe, squared toe, rounded toe. Leather, snakeskin, ostrich skin. His and hers. Johnny Cash sings "When the Man Comes Around" over the store speakers. A matronly, no-nonsense saleswoman who knows what's what takes me in hand, and within twenty minutes I'm walking out in my new boots.

"You don't want a pair?" I ask my friend.

"Haven't worn cowboy boots in thirty years."

Over at Dickies, the ten-thousand-seat arena is packed. We take our seats one row below the rafters just as a local pastor is blessing the event. This is followed by the Pledge of Allegiance, followed in turn by the National Anthem, and then, since Lockheed Martin F-16 and F-35s are built nearby, the sound effect of fighter jets roaring past at close quarters in what is known locally as "the Sound of Freedom," and the rodeo is set to begin.

There's the roping competition, in which two men on horses chase a steer, one ropes the horns, the other the feet. Whichever team does this the fastest wins. Steer wrestling entails getting the horned animal to the ground, barehanded, then tying its hooves. More than one competitor is kicked hard, sometimes in the head. And of course there is bull riding, in which a cowboy is placed on the back of a gargantuan and unhappy bull and tries to hold on for eight seconds without getting his spine snapped or worse.

There is an announcer narrating all of this over the loudspeaker, offering a kind of play-by-play commentary in the style of a football game. He is half as funny as he thinks he is. All of this is more exciting and entertaining than either Eddie or I anticipated. When the women on horseback race ferociously around a series of strategically placed barrels trying to beat the clock, the announcer hails the "little ladies'" efforts. But what really gets Eddie's attention is the mutton busting.

A child of five, wearing a helmet, is placed prone on the back of a sheep, wraps his arms and legs around the animal's torso, and holds on for dear life until the darting sheep flings the child from its back.

One youngster after another is sent airborne within seconds. Most bounce up quickly after being dislodged. There's something oddly amusing about this sight, if it weren't for the fact that these are small children being trampled like rag dolls.

Eddie is flabbergasted. "Two words," he says in disbelief. "Child abuse!" We watch as a young girl—the only girl in the competition—clings tight until the far end of the ring, sealing the win and delighting the crowd. Eddie throws up his hands.

"We ban *Diary of Anne Frank* in school, but we let five-year-old kids get their heads kicked in riding a sheep? What the fuck is happening to America?"

After such wholesome pleasures, by the next morning Eddie is ready for some action.

"Shreveport, my friend," he says between bites of biscuit at the R&K II.

"I just came from Louisiana."

"But you weren't with the master."

"Oh, no."

"That's right, my young amigo… wait for it…"

"Please don't."

"Can you say… 'snake eyes'?"

And we're on I-20 heading east. Since Eddie is driving, I have no issue with plowing over the interstate for three hours. And since Eddie is excited about the prospect of shooting craps, he drives very fast. We pass a billboard that advises "Pray to God," then another that asks, "Who is Jesus?" Eddie mentions a cholesterol-lowering drug he's begun taking, and then a website that matches older men with money and young women who desire to be "kept."

Eddie's adolescent cackle rings out. "Can you imagine a worse idea?"

We're not actually going to Shreveport, but its sister city across the Red River, Bossier City. Once the site of an oil boom, before that a railroad town, and earlier still a cotton exporting river landing, today Bossier City's raison d'être is its half dozen casinos. With close to 70,000 inhabitants, it is said to be the fastest-growing city in Louisiana—but the Las Vegas strip it is not.

When we check in to the Horseshoe Casino, the man behind the desk with glasses and toupee looks closely at my license and reads out, "McCarthy." He pronounces the name correctly. Then, "You related to Paul?"

I've actually heard this question before.

"That's McCart-NEY," I say, overenunciating for emphasis. "I'm McCarTHY."

The man continues to stare at me, his eyes still questioning.

"They're cousins," Eddie says from over my shoulder, just to move things along.

Impressed, the man nods and hands me a plastic room keycard.

Back at the start of this extended cross-country trip I didn't know I'd be taking, while in Atlantic City, I stopped by the roulette table in Caesar's and placed $5 on number thirty-five black. There was a reason for this.

When we were all younger and stupider and living in New York, during one of our not infrequent runs to Atlantic City, Eddie, Seve, and I had blown all our money save the price of a final drink and the toll fare home. We sat at the casino bar staring up at the television at an old Abbott and Costello movie. The two comedians were in a casino, just as we were. Costello stood beside a roulette wheel and someone asked how old he was. He replied, "Thirty-five." The croupier, hearing this, called out, "Thirty-five for the fat man" and pushed Lou's money over to the number. The number came in.

Seeing this, we three stooges rose from the bar in unison and stumbled to the roulette table. "A sign from the gods," Eddie proclaimed. He then slapped down our toll money on number thirty-five. "Money plays," he confidently told the croupier. The wheel spun. Round and round it went. The silver ball came to land on number 2.

We blew through the tolls home, didn't get arrested, and considered ourselves winners. Every time any of us have been in a casino since that day we have placed a bet on number thirty-five. It has never come in.

Now as Eddie and I enter the casino, we head directly to the roulette wheel without discussing the matter. Eddie places a $5 chip on number thirty-five. The wheel spins. Neither of us speaks. The ball bounces. We lean forward. It settles on number sixteen. We turn our backs and walk toward the craps table.

"My garden needs to grooowww." Eddie rattles his green chips from one hand to the other.

I watch as he wins and loses at the craps table and then wins and loses some more. I place a few bets on the pass line, but having never really understood craps and preferring blackjack, I'm content to mostly watch. By midnight Eddie's about even. We retire to the lone open restaurant. There's a couple, both in mobility scooters, at a table across the room eating pancakes and drinking large sodas. The place has the stale, recirculated air that fuels the forced hope and denied exhaustion typical of casinos in the middle of a timeless night.

The waiter offers us a drink. When he retreats, Eddie wonders if I'm ever tempted by alcohol. I stopped drinking decades earlier, after drowning much of the blossom of my youth under a waterfall of booze. He's the only one of my friends who ever openly wonders about this.

I shrug. "I've kind of been placed in a position of neutrality around it," I say. "But as any good drunk will tell you, 'All bets are off for tomorrow.'"

My friend nods, satisfied.

I chew some of the ice in my water glass. "Have you ever thought that gambling is Alzheimer's avoidant behavior?"

Eddie looks up from his burger.

"All the fast counting and figuring," I explain.

Eddie considers. "That is a very good point, my brother." Which then leads him to the obvious conclusion—"See, gambling is good for you."

Returning to the topic that set all this in motion, I ask Eddie why he thinks we're friends.

"Probably our similarities," he says.

Strange, but I never considered us all that similar. I certainly emulated him in my youth, but that's different.

Eddie goes on. "We have complex things in common. It's almost genetic. We just have a brother thing. When you can communicate and not have to talk, that says something."

"What about our not really talking for years?" I ask.

"None of us talked near as much when we were in the throes of raising kids. But to go five, ten years without talking and pick up…that speaks to something. It also connects you to your youth. We're foundational relationships for each other. That's significant." He sips his Dr Pepper. "This is a team sport."

It's the kind of conversation that happens easily in the middle of the night in a place designed to exist without past or future. When the check is placed on the table, Eddie's tired face looks across at me.

"Shall we go ensure some brain function?"

Back at the craps table Eddie gets on a roll, and the late night allows a boldness on my part. I begin to play the field line. Eddie instructs me on some more sophisticated "place" and "buy" bets.

The croupier, with whom Eddie has been carrying on a running conversation, asks, "Teaching your friend some bad habits?"

Eddie smiles, reaching to collect his winnings. "Oh, that's all I've taught him."

Austin, Texas

The final tally shows me winning several hundred dollars—the result of beginner's luck on the craps table. Eddie lost a few hundred. "I had planned to lose five hundred, so I'm a winner," he boasts. After beating it back to Cleburne under the cover of night, we say our goodbyes—Eddie has an early meeting tomorrow in Dallas. Our reconnection has been as uncomplicated, playful, and as quickly intimate as I could have hoped.

In the morning, I return to the R&K Café II. I'm thinking about pancakes. The large room is half full. Carhartt and mesh caps. T-shirts and tattoos. After I order my short stack, an email from Don arrives—as it typically does—a few days after mine to him. It reads, simply, *Mississippi? Texas?! Where next?*

Without taking myself seriously, I type, *Oakland??* and send.

Don and I met fifteen years ago. We were teamed together by a publisher to edit a book of travel essays. Don was a legend in the field of travel writing, while I was considered by many to be an interloper. We met for lunch in New York to discuss the possibility and instantly hit it off. We did the book together—meaning Don did the lion's share of the work and my name went first on the cover. And a friendship grew. He's a genuine, tender, and buoyant spirit. We tend to laugh a lot when we get together, which is infrequently.

My pancakes arrive, and while I'm spreading some whipped butter on top, an uncharacteristically rapid reply comes in from Don. *YES!!! I'm here for three weeks till I go to Paris. Come on out!*

I smile, but Oakland is a long way.

Then, while pouring syrup, I type into my phone, *Driving distance from Cleburne Tx to Oakland Ca.*

1,700 miles.

And that's on major interstates.

"Whoa," I say aloud, dismissing the notion.

While eating, my mind drifts to things that need doing once I'm back home. And then without knowing exactly when I made the decision to stand up, I'm walking out to the car to retrieve my Rand McNally Road Atlas. Back inside, I push my half-eaten pancakes to the edge of the table and spread the large map out.

I mean, if I did go, I wouldn't be traveling on the interstates. So just how far is it...

Once I've begun this type of thinking, I know what's happening—it will only take me another cup of tea to accept the idea.

I ask my waitress for some more hot water.

My friendships with Seve, Matthew, and Eddie are—as Eddie aptly labeled them—foundational relationships. While nothing can replace those early connections, friends made later in life have rich value if for no other reason than that it can be so much more difficult to make friends as we get older. They require a conscious and active (and vulnerable-making) commitment in the way those early friendships did not, when friendship seemed to "just happen." And they can propel us into our future in a way those longtime friendships don't necessarily. The lack of history with newer friends can promote feelings of expansion—a fresh, outside perspective can prove liberating.

Paying my bill at the register, my spirits soar not only at the idea of seeing Don, but of continuing along the open road, on this unorthodox exploration of friendship with the men I've been meeting along the way. When the cashier hands me my change, she suggests that I "have a blessed day."

In a fashion that's consistent with the improvisational, indirect, maybe even ridiculous nature of this trip, I head off toward Northern California by pointing due south. On a journey of thousands of miles with long hours behind the wheel, the three hours from Cleburne to Austin is close enough for it to be justified as "in the neighborhood." I'm headed that way because I've suddenly got a date there with two Texans for some Mexican food.

Some time ago I'd read journalist Lawrence Wright's book, *God Save Texas*. In it, he spoke movingly of his close friendship with a fellow writer, Stephen Harrigan. Wright and I have a mutual friend. So, while I sat in the R&K finishing my tea, I reached out. And in the kind of serendipity and aligning of stars that go a long way in justifying this kind of escapade (at least to the person doing it), the two men are in town and agree to meet me on very short notice.

I head south out of town on two-lane State Route 174, following a green pickup for forty miles. In tiny Crawford, neither local resident George W. Bush nor anyone else is out and about. A freight train pulling hundreds of cars tracks my progress along the two-lane Lone Star Parkway, then once past charmless McGregor, it's ninety more miles to Austin.

It's in the back booth of Julio's restaurant near High Park in North Austin that I encounter the two friends. Stephen is bald with a genial face covered by a trim beard and round glasses. Lawrence looks like he could have been cast as an altar boy or a Cub Scout more than a half century earlier—except for the occasional inquisitor's glare in his blue eyes. The two share a long history. Both were born in the same hospital in Oklahoma City. Both moved to Texas as small children. Without knowing, they went to grade school across the street from each other in Abilene at the same time. When they met in 1979, both drove the same type of car, each used the same brand of infant car seat, and in 1980 their friendship began in earnest when they were both hired to write for *Texas Monthly* magazine. It's a bond that's continued uninterrupted ever since. They live around the corner from each other not far from this dive.

Larry, as he prefers to be called, sips iced tea and lemonade and considers my question of just exactly what it was that drew them to each other.

"When we first met, Steve and I recognized ourselves in each other. Our quest was very similar. There are a lot of people you know, but there are only a few you deeply identify with."

Steve, who presents more like an East Coast college professor than a Texan, has been nodding along with his friend's remarks. "Five or six times in your life, if you're lucky, you'll meet somebody who you just really connect with. Often those connections are broken by time or circumstance but, in the case of Larry and me, we've been in the same place all this time."

"But Steve has a wide range of friends and is a much better friend to others than I am."

"I would say exactly the opposite." Steve leans back.

"He's wrong." Larry leans in on his elbows. As is frequently the case with these two, Larry takes the lead, although Steve often has the last, considered word.

"I was talking to one of my daughters," Steve says, "about the difference between male and female friendships. Being the father of three girls I can tell you that they're always checking in on the status of their friendships. It's an active conversation. 'How we doing?' But we don't talk about that. I don't know that we'd have the vocabulary or the interest to talk about it. It's just there."

"You ever fight?" I ask.

"No, but we've thought about it." Larry grins.

I smile at what sounds like the well-worn line of an old married couple. "Are you competitive?" I ask.

"Kind of sort of," Steve says.

"We've written the same number of books," Larry says.

"You're one ahead of me now, I think," Steve corrects him.

"Maybe not competitive, but we're keeping track," Larry says.

"Ambition can be a problem for some friendships because it leads to competition, but it can also be a bonding force, because you're with people who are following the same road, looking for the same elusive destination—into the rainbow. You're on a journey." Steve glances toward his friend. "But increasingly we're sort of satisfied in the part of the world we inhabit."

"I don't know," Larry says. "A while ago you told me, 'I'm still trying to make it.' And I feel the same way."

"So do I," I say. "But I'm starting to get to the point where I don't care if I make it."

"And then as you move past sixty you'll feel more and more that way," Steve says. "But the ambition is still there. It's not the same kind of ambition. It's more personal maybe. You're kind of aware of what your horizon is and that ambition exists for self-respect or self-exploration, so you keep at it."

Larry has been staring out the window, considering. "And then when you get even older there's this sense of being in a life raft. You're surrounded by death, your classmates are dying"—he turns to Steve—"and here we are still on this raft. So, there's this added connection between us because of our age and what we're facing. We think about that a lot. I don't talk to very many people about the complications that age brings and the anxiety that comes with it. But Steve and I talk about it all the time. It presumes a level of intimacy that you don't normally have with other friends, where if you start to express something about your anxiety about mortality, then you're opening yourself up to pity, derision, or false responses that are probably even worse. We know where we stand with each other."

Steve, as he often does during our talk, takes his friend's remarks into account and places them into a kind of gentle, macro perspective. "We've been talking shop all our lives, so talking mortality and illness, it's just an extension of that shop talk. It's just practical."

To prove that point, the personal talk turns to shop talk. "Steve is the best editor I've ever had. He understands where you're going with it and why you fell short. When I finished *The Looming Tower*, I sent it to Steve before anyone, before my editor, and the first thing Steve said was 'You gotta take that *New Yorker* magazine voice out of it.' So, I went through it again taking that formality out of it. I don't know that I could have received that from anyone else. It's not a master or teacher relationship. It's a 'two guys talking' relationship."

"How rare is male friendship anyway?" Steve sounds a bit incredulous. "I mean is there fundamentally a deficiency in the male psyche that prevents it?"

Before I can answer with details of my own atrophied relations, Larry jumps in. "My dad didn't have friends, except in the military. Only once did I meet any of his friends, on a fishing trip to Wyoming."

This hits me like a slap upside the head. Not actively pursuing and maintaining my own friendships, neither my long-distance ones nor those closer to home, has not only diminished my personal experiences but diminished me as a parent. When Sam said to me, "You don't really have any friends, do you, Dad?" he not only set in motion this cross-country folly but unwittingly illuminated a failing of mine as his father. It's an accepted truism that kids don't learn by what we say, but by the behavior we model for them. My lack of active engagement with friends, my withdrawal, has set a poor example. It's been a loss, not just for me but for my children.

These two, on the other hand, can feel so close as to almost meld, or at least confuse things. Partnering on a project for Hollywood once, they went to meet Jane Fonda. As the door opened, Fonda greeted them, "Hi, I'm Jane."

Reaching for her proffered hand, Larry said, "I'm Steve Harrigan."

To which Steve said, "No you're not. I'm Steve Harrigan."

After that, Fonda was never able to keep the two straight. The project never happened.

Yet seeing the closeness of these two, one doesn't so much complete the other—as is often stated about intimate marriages—

but enhances the other. I wonder aloud what would be lost from their lives if the other weren't in it.

"We were talking about Austin one time, and I said that if Steve died, I'd probably leave," Larry says matter-of-factly.

"That kind of statement certainly demonstrates this friendship is a massive priority," I say.

"Well"—Larry gets the gleam in his eye—"I haven't tested that theory. He's still alive."

"This friendship is going to end when one of us dies," Steve says simply. "But if you're asking if we had never had each other, that's a big thing to consider. First, I would have had a wildly different career. But I would have had a smaller life. I wouldn't have had an example to follow, a peer, and that companionship and the confidence that came with that. I would have been a completely different person."

"As I started this conversation," Larry says. "Our friendship has been about recognizing in someone else something of ourselves."

This feels similar to what Eddie was referring to in the casino late at night—when he talked about our "similarities," that our connection was "almost genetic."

Larry goes on. "And that feels utterly normal. Friendship is not intense. It's normal."

"This may be the first conversation we've had about our friendship." Steve is suddenly bemused. "It's routine, it's habit, it's a need you didn't know you had in a way you didn't know you needed."

Without my noticing, the chairs around us have been upended and put on tabletops, and the floor is being swept. Larry asks if I'd like to continue our conversation back at his house, a few minutes' drive away. I follow his black Mercedes to an upscale suburb and park in front when he turns into the driveway of a large stone house. Inside the den, Larry's wife, Roberta, is at a corner table doing a jigsaw puzzle. She receives us graciously and returns to her puzzle. Steve sits on the couch while Larry and I each take up overstuffed chairs. Our conversation picks right up, and I ask if friendship in general has been a priority in their lives.

"No," Larry says, putting one of his cowboy boots up on the coffee table. "I've always been mystified where friendship comes from. I had friends in high school, but we were outcasts, and we didn't keep up those relationships."

I think of my own long-abandoned high school friends. "Outcasts rarely do," I say.

Larry considers me a moment. "There's this quote, I can't remember who said it, 'Friendship is only possible among good people.'"

"Cicero," Roberta says without looking up from her jigsaw puzzle.

"Cicero, right. Thanks." Larry nods toward his wife. "You can argue with that proposition but, if you're in a friendship, you have to have the qualities that can support a friendship."

"What are those qualities?" I ask.

Larry considers, "Loyalty, and truth telling, and patience, and forgiveness, and humor."

I look to Steve.

He nods. "That's a pretty good list."

Austin, Texas
Part 2

A few years ago, I met two young men named Ryan and Chris. They were at a public water fountain on the side of the road outside Pamplona, Spain. I was with my son Sam—who was quick to dub them "The Boys." We were all near the beginning of a five-hundred-mile walk across the north of Spain on the Camino de Santiago, an ancient pilgrimage route. Over the course of the next month, Sam and I would lose and reunite with The Boys numerous times, forging a connection that is typical of, and feels unique to, such a perspective-altering experience as the Camino. The Boys had an obvious bond and playful sense of fellowship. They also live in Austin. So I call them.

"I'm meeting Chris for brunch," Ryan shouts to me over the phone. "I'll change the reservation to a better place. Join us!"

I find a place to park near the Tecovas boot shop on South Congress Avenue, one of Austin's buzziest thoroughfares. It's on streets like this, walking past bars and trendy shops, heavy with young and attractive foot traffic, that I quickly conclude after a two-minute assessment, "I should live here."

I meet up with Ryan walking into the restaurant where he's made our reservation. It's a more upscale, white-tablecloth place than I know he can comfortably afford. Rake thin with a trim beard, Ryan is deceptively accessible. Chris, a St. Bernard of a man, with a broad grin and a wide-open manner suffused with an ever-so-elusive quality, is a few minutes late, as usual. Both are barely thirty. Both have winning personalities.

I learned some of their origin story in Spain, but I get more here. They met in 2018, both patients at a drug and alcohol rehab facility in Colorado.

"I remember seeing you," Chris says, looking at Ryan across the table, "and thinking, I'm not gonna get along with this guy."

We all laugh.

"Well, I probably wasn't the most likable guy in the world back then."

"None of us were," Chris says, coming to the aid of his friend in a way that's typical of these two.

"We were doing one of those rehab exercises where you had to go put your hand on the shoulder of someone you felt a connection with," Ryan remembers, laughing. "I had just gotten there and didn't know anyone, but I went up to you and just put my hand on your shoulder."

"And I remember thinking," Chris takes over the story, "'Oh, uh, okay.' And I guess that was kind of it."

After rehab the two moved on to a sober living facility, then to an even more unstructured home. There were relapses and restarts, moments of living in cars. Ryan crashed on Chris's couch for months.

"There's something to be said for getting sober together. It's a different type of friendship than anything I've ever experienced," Chris says. "We were feeding off each other. We wanted to get better. We wanted our lives to get bigger. And at some point, we were going in this new direction together. It was real. Even though there have been relapses, that's just a piece of what's happened. The foundation was set. We've been able to come back and grow our lives."

"It's definitely a thing that holds you together more so than, say, a work colleague," Ryan says.

Chris agrees. "Seeing someone get well is something beautiful, getting well alongside someone is a powerful bonding experience. There's a richness to the connection. There've been times when he's almost been dead, and moments when I've almost been dead…"

They both nod, and we sit with that for a moment.

"Remember when I called you on that Christmas Eve?" Chris starts again, as if recalling a happy evening around the fire.

Ryan laughs. "You were like, 'Hey, man, I'm polishing off beer number eighteen.' And I was just like, 'How's that going for you?'"

"There's no judgment," Chris says. "That's the thing."

"I feel that I can tell him anything," Ryan says. "That if anything happens, I have this person I can lean on, truly. There are a lot of people who are my friends, but I just wouldn't feel comfortable or, or… comforted in the same way as I do by this man."

Each has a relationship with the other's parents. "When I've been bad, he talks to my dad, and when he's been in a bad way, his mom calls me," Ryan says.

"We would have been friends in high school if we'd known each other, but the recovery aspect has been the cornerstone," Chris sums up. "And he's supported me through all the spiritual stuff I've done."

"Yeah," Ryan says. "Four years ago, when you went on that vision quest thing, the sweat lodge." Ryan turns to me. "And he calls me up and asks me to come."

"I guess I thought you might get something out of it. Like I did. That you're seeking, like me."

"What are you seeking?" I ask.

Both pause.

"To fill the void," Chris says, in a grappling nonchalant fashion that captures his contradictions.

"Seeking what my heart is trying to tell me," Ryan says. "So many people look for their answer in money. But with him, there's this unspoken understanding that none of that truly matters. That we're looking for something else. And to know that he feels that way too is huge. What's important is a connection with people and living a path that tries to open you up to what your heart is telling you, not relying on monetary things to fill that."

Chris is quick to jump in. "Not that I don't want that. There are days when I feel behind everybody. But when I really stop and think about it, I'm grateful and wouldn't change a thing."

"The Camino is a spiritual exercise for many people," I say, revisiting our shared past. "It certainly was for me, and I think for my son as well—"

Before I can finish my thought, Ryan jumps in. "I'd always wanted to do it, and I needed something more to hold on to than just some recovery job."

"Yeah," Chris adds, "he called me up and said, 'I'm gonna walk across Spain,' and I just said, 'I'm gonna come with you.' I didn't even ask. And that was it."

The Boys laugh. "A lot of people say they're gonna do stuff, and this motherfucker actually did," Ryan says with admiration.

"And?" I ask.

"For me," Ryan says, "however cheesy it sounds, it showed that anything is possible."

Chris nods. "It opened a door."

Uvalde, Texas

Leaving The Boys and their hard-earned hope, I head straight into darkness. All day the Texas sky has been stifled by a shroud of unyielding gray. Then, on US Route 57, a faint sliver of blue becomes visible at the distant vanishing point ahead. Then a fireball sun, too big to squeeze between the horizon and the clouds, drops slowly, exposing itself piece by piece. When it's gone, light reflects up onto the sea of clouds and displaces the dull gray with florid red. Driving directly into this, I strain to keep focus on the two-lane road. Large trucks sporadically come at me and roar past, sending a shudder through the car. Slowly, slowly, the light in the sky begins to die. I take small comfort in its refusal to yield—it's a full hour before it loses life entirely. By then the consolation I took in its determination has surrendered to a kind of dread. The night, when it finally falls fully, falls hard and complete. Only the high beams of occasional trucks coming directly at me, and then the woosh and the shaking of the car, break the solitude. I harbor an irrational fear that just as each truck is almost upon me, I will suffer a tire blowout and my car will careen over the line and smash into the oncoming eighteen-wheeler. I had wanted to be at my destination by nightfall.

I turn north on Route 140, and Seve calls.

"I'm surprised the call went through," I say by way of greeting. "I'm in the middle of fucking nowhere."

I tell him about the sky and where I'm headed.

"Mmm," he groans. "Why you going there?"

"I don't know," I tell him.

"I wish I was th—" But the call cuts out.

In Uvalde, I make a left on Main Street and then a left onto South Grove, another left on Geraldine Street, and then pull to a stop at the corner of Old Carrizo Road. To my right, under the glow of a streetlamp, twenty-one small white crosses have been placed on the sidewalk in front of Robb Elementary School to honor those murdered here.

On May 24, 2022, a gunman with an assault rifle climbed the fence onto school property and began shooting. He then entered the building via the northwest door, turned right down the hallway, and walked into connecting rooms 111 and 112. There he gunned down nineteen fourth-grade children and two teachers.

Police were alerted before the killer had entered school property. (He had taken shots at two people across the street, who immediately called 911.) After rushing to the scene and even entering the building, the police then took no steps to stop the shooter for seventy-seven minutes. Their inaction brought shame upon them, stoked outrage throughout the country, and compounded the heartache of an already unimaginable tragedy.

I get out and approach the homemade shrine. The names of the victims have been handwritten on the crosses. I read each of them. Small stuffed animals have been left, plastic flowers, bracelets, notes have been scrawled, photos are taped up. There's a baseball. The low-slung brick building is dark behind a temporary wire fence. Its windows are black. An orange tabby cat approaches and stops when he sees me. We look at each other. He darts off, low to the ground.

As I'm ready to leave, from the darkness of the driveway of the building, the running lights of a car I hadn't noticed snap on. I start. As my eyes adjust, I see it's a police car. Perhaps it's just my nerves, but the gesture feels aggressive. Am I being sent a signal to move along? The car takes no further action. The lights remain lit. There's no one else around. In some form of protest, in anger, I remain where I am for a long time.

"There are still grudges," Ben, a heavyset guy in his thirties, tells me the following morning in the Local Fix coffee shop. "There're still hard feelings, the way it was handled. Can you imagine your child in there? And they did nothing."

"I have a ten-year-old boy in the fourth grade," I say.

"What's his name?"

"Rowan."

"I still see parents wearing those T-shirts they had made, 'In Memory of…' People say you have to move on. How do you move on from that?"

"Has the town healed at all?"

"No." Ben shakes his head. "People don't talk about it. Not unless there's a reporter here."

Originally from Waller, Texas, Ben recently got engaged and is moving away. "Either to Colorado or South Dakota. The people, the town, it's not as nice as it was."

"You have friends here you'll miss?"

"Used to have good friends. Doesn't really feel that way anymore."

Over at the Broadway 830 pizza joint on Main Street, Rosa tells me a similar story. "We used to just run around everywhere when we were kids, but now…" Her voice trails off. "I got three small cousins; they've never been the same."

There are a few signs around town, in storefront windows and on billboards, "UVALDE STRONG," and I see one that says, "Pray for Uvalde."

I return to Robb Elementary in the daylight. I walk around to the back of the school. Swing sets and monkey bars stand idle in the overgrown yard. A police cruiser sits in the parking lot, its door flung open. I read the names of the victims on the crosses again. A couple from San Antonio arrive. We exchange greetings. I yield the space to them and return to my car and watch as they take in the shrine. They look, then stare off, then wander without direction and then return to the crosses. They appear bewildered, helpless—the same way I feel sitting behind the wheel.

Dolores calls.

"Why are you there?" she asks.

I give her the same answer I gave Seve. "I don't know."

We're silent for a moment.

"To bear witness?" she asks.

"It just feels important somehow."

Travel for me, the best of travel, has never been about beaches or bucket lists, or even about having a good time, but about exactly what Dolores said—seeing for myself, bearing witness. And through that, trying to place myself in the context of my larger surroundings and the wider world. Yet I, like so many, am incapable of reconciling an atrocity like Uvalde.

An online "friend" of the shooter's, who said the two "talked on a daily basis" on the social media site Yubo, described an angry person who was always arguing with people but at other times appeared emotionless.[1] A former girlfriend said he was "lonely and depressed." CNN described the shooter as "a loner" and someone "with few if any friends"[2]—conditions that could describe many, yet seem almost cliché for people who commit such atrocities.

I set out on this trip to combat my own encroaching sensation of separateness that I felt was beginning to impinge on my life, to limit my experiences. Quietude seeping toward isolation was beginning to limit the vista of my experiences. Yet the summits of aloneness and disconnection, the peaks of isolation and alienation that the shooter reached defeat my imagining.

"You want to talk to Rowan?" my wife asks me.

"Yes."

Eagle Pass, Texas

Farm-to-Market Road 481 takes me southwest out of Uvalde. A dozen miles from the border with Mexico, I take up two-lane Highway 57 and see my first Border Patrol SUV, white with a green stripe. It's parked by the side of the road, pointed into the desert of scrub and cactus. Whoever is coming over this despairing expanse of earth on foot is in dire need.

Eagle Pass, on the banks of the Rio Grande, has at times strained under the weight of not only migration but the political microscope that's been trained upon it. Cast as the poster child for failed immigration policy, it's been depicted as a dangerous, lawless mess, overrun with the undocumented streaming in, willing to do anything to get through La Puerta de Mexico.

Any border town is a place of transience, of curt exchanges, callousness, need—Eagle Pass is no exception. The pangs of desperation are not far beneath the surface of any encounter. It is a transactional place, a place one could easily come to grief. There is little to recommend it other than the two bridges that are its reason for being.

I approach International Bridge #1 on foot. It's a two-lane affair with pedestrian walkways on either side, one for going, one for coming. At the dirty window before the turnstile, I'm asked for $1. I pay the officer and then wait, assuming there must be more to do, but am told in a hissing tone, "Go on, go on."

The US-bound traffic on the bridge is bumper-to-bumper across its entire expanse. There is no outbound traffic. The bridge extends over a primitive golf course with men in brightly colored shirts trudging over blistered grass. Approaching the river, three rows of barbed wire backed by a long string of shipping containers are visible deterrents. The Rio Grande is narrower than I expected. There is no activity on the brown water. Leading up from the river on the Mexican side is an unguarded, gentle dirt bank. Once in Mexico, I walk through an outdated metal detector and am waved on. No one in either country has asked to see any form of identification.

Piedras Negras is the Mexican mirror version of Eagle Pass. Charm is elusive. I'm alternately invisible and eyed with disinterested suspicion. Along Calle Ocampo, a dog pants in the shade outside a barbershop. A vendor sells cheap flip-flops on the broken sidewalk. Inside El Patio bar, Mexican pop music blares. With no windows, the only light is provided by the spill from the open door and a sky-blue laser raking the air. Three old men are sitting separately on high stools sipping Tecate in longneck bottles. My Mexican Coke, sweetened with cane sugar and not the corn syrup found in American Cokes, is delicious.

I wander for another hour, consider a taco from a street vendor, and return to the bridge. After being asked to pay US thirty cents, I'm nodded through. Halfway across the bridge, directly above the river, at a plaque delineating the border separating Mexico from the US, three border guards sit on stools chatting.

"Got your document on you?" the officer with a goatee asks. He doesn't seem to care that much. I reach into my pocket, and before I can extract any kind of proof, he says, "Perfect, thank you."

Once back in America, I wait behind a Mexican mother and a young girl as their papers are inspected. I go to offer up my ID and am waved through. My skin color gives me a free pass.

My experience in Eagle Pass is not one overlaid with a sense of imminent or even lurking peril. The apparent laissez-faire manner of all my interactions surprises and then relaxes me. But in time, the seemingly casual nature of these encounters emerges as something else. Buying toothpaste in a 99-cent store, it dawns on me that what I initially perceived to be a palatable patina cast by offhanded apathy is more accurately viewed as weary disregard for the basic value and nobility of life. And when pressed, such indifference permits otherwise unacceptable behavior to be passed off without second thought, without need for justification.

I track the border northwest on Route 277, then pick up Route 90. Once over the badly depleted Amistad Reservoir, an inspection station forces me off the road. An immigration officer glances first in my back seat and then at me. He says something I don't understand.

"Sorry?" I say.

"Are you a US citizen?" the officer enunciates with exaggerated politeness.

"Oh, sorry. Yes. I am."

He manages a tight smile, but the snap of his wrist as he waves me on betrays a disdain I don't feel I've entirely earned.

Comstock, Texas

I find unlikely relief in the town of Comstock, twenty miles up the road. The word "town" is too grand a term for humble Comstock, with a population of 159. Its single-pump gas station, lone bar, and motel offer little inducement to slow, let alone stop. How many times have I passed such places with unquestioning dismissal—if I've considered them at all. But I've had enough for one day and turn in to the motel parking lot. Mine is the only car.

There are several small water bowls on the ground by the entrance, and the half dozen underfed cats nearby scatter as I walk up. Several take refuge under my car and peer out at me. Entering the small office, I encounter clothes thrown over the back of the chair behind a counter strewn with papers. There are a few empty Pepsi bottles, and a small bell. A shotgun with a high-powered scope is propped up in the corner. Through a closed door, I hear shouting. I ring the bell several times, trying to get my timing right, between shouts, so the ding of the bell can be heard. Eventually, I do, and a bearded man with a red MAGA hat pokes his nose out. He's on the phone. "I gotta go, I gotta go," he barks into the receiver and puts it down. This is Shawn. To go with his hat, Shawn wears a T-shirt with the Lone Star on the chest that reads, "TAKE BACK AUSTIN." On its back is printed: "Info Wars."

"You got a reservation?" Shawn snaps.

Noting the empty parking lot, I ask, "Do I need one?"

"I got plenty a rooms." His tone softens. "It's eighty-eight dollars."

It seems steep, but it's the only show in town. "I'll pay you cash," I tell him.

"Just give me eighty then," Shawn says. "And you can sign the register if you want."

"Do you need me to?"

He shakes his head. "Just gimme the money." Then, digging for a key—"You're in room two."

"Who's in one?"

"Nobody. Storage."

"That's not a Texas accent," I say.

"No, sir, southeast Kentucky."

Shawn came to this lonely spot in western Texas nine years ago.

"Mind if I ask why?"

"I don't mind. I like talkin'. I had me an accident. I was tyin' a bull rope to an old oak tree, and it snapped. That thing shoved my pinkie and next two fingers back up into my hand." He holds his left hand aloft for me to see.

"Ouch," I say.

"My mom and dad—they're gone now—they were here and they suggested I come down. They needed my help anyway." Shawn pauses long enough to take a breath and continues. "I done already had my family and I'm proud of 'em, but I don't want no more. I'm happy on my own. So…" He scratches under his hat, then starts up again. "I'm here for a reason. I'm not proud, but I ain't ashamed or embarrassed about nothing neither. It's my fault where I'm at in life. I do what I gotta do where I'm at till I can do better. Then I'll get home."

Unsure about the specifics of what Shawn is talking about, the weight of his burden feels clear. I receive him with a nod.

Shawn walks me down to my room to show me its intricacies—where the light switch is, the faucet, the television. And he's proud to show me the "pavilion" out back. It's a corrugated metal roof over a poured cement floor in the rear of the parking lot. There's a barbecue and an ice chest. "You can have a party here if you want, just not in the room," Shawn says.

"I'm on my own," I tell him.

"Suit yourself."

There's a tenderness about Shawn that belies initial impressions.

I wonder if there are many parties in the pavilion and if friends are easy to come by in such a quiet spot.

"Easy as peasy. Just say 'Hi, it's hot today,' and go from there."

"It wasn't hot today."

"I was demonstrating, Andy."

"Sorry."

Shawn stops in the parking lot and clarifies. "The way I was raised was to just be as good to a stranger as to my brother. That is if they let you. Lot of people won't let you get close. I'll holler out to anybody, but some folks don't like that."

A small tabby cat scurries over and rubs against Shawn's ankle. Shawn falls silent for the first time. Then reaches down and scratches behind the cat's ear.

"I'm around a lot of people, I interact with a lot of numbers. But"—he shrugs—"I ain't got too many close friends here."

"It is pretty quiet," I say.

Shawn nods, stares off for a moment, then repeats, "I'll get home."

I want to say something more, but I'm not sure what. A dry wind blows.

"Hey." Shawn brightens. "Want to see my rock garden?"

"You bet," I say.

Under the motel sign out front are a bunch of stones covering an area of maybe ten feet by five, clustered together like a kidney-shaped pool. In the middle of the grouping is an overturned green bucket. Resting on top of the bucket is a rock with a smiley face crudely painted on it. "He's my gardener," Sean explains. "Made it myself."

No one would leave home with the intention to drive thousands of miles to find themselves here, yet staring down at the upturned bucket and painted rock, I experience an unlikely feeling of solidarity with Shawn. If friendship is, as the writer James Baldwin said, "the work of mirroring and magnifying each other's light," then for this moment at least, Shawn and I are friends. The sudden tenderness, the unguarded vulnerability of Shawn's light has touched mine and lifted the darkness that's hung over me since Uvalde and Eagle Pass.

"Thanks for showing me this, Shawn."

"Thanks for looking, Andy."

Across the street, at the J&P Bar and Grill, three young men in stained work clothes and dirty boots sit at a table, dividing their attention between the college basketball game on TV and their phones. None of them speak. When the food arrives, they eat in silence. By contrast, three young women at the bar chat and laugh often with the female bartender.

While I'm eating the best cheeseburger I've had on the road, the bar's owner cautions me to fill my tank as it's ninety miles to the next…anything. We talk baseball, and Texas. Simple connection can arrive in the most unlikely places, and I pass a memorably inconsequential evening.

Back across the road at the motel, I sit outside my door and watch the moon rise over the wire fence across the parking lot. A BMW motorcycle has appeared in my absence. A large man with ginger hair and beard, Carl, now inhabits room 3. Carl has a lot on his mind. "I got a big decision to make in the next forty-eight hours. I gotta go left or right, so I came out here to ride, think it over."

"Is that how you usually make those kinds of decisions?" I ask.

"I let the road talk to me. I just ride."

I hear pride in Carl's description of his process. Such lone wolf philosophy strikes me as distinctly male, and a typically American idea of what it is to be a man, fulfilling a notion of rugged individualism, strength, and solitude. We chat amiably, me in the chair I've pulled out, my foot propped up on the pillar supporting the overhanging roof, him fiddling with his bike, until there is no light left in the sky.

In my room I flip on the TV, and *True Grit*, the John Wayne movie, is on. I laugh. There is perhaps no one who did more to propagate the stoic, macho version of American manhood than Wayne. I watch for a few minutes. His brand of masculinity seems so silly, so outdated, so limited, and yet it lingers in the psyche of men—men like Carl. And me.

In youth, precisely because I didn't possess this hardened, stolid exterior, I harbored an insecurity that I wasn't man enough, that I was somehow insufficient. That I didn't aspire to such a hardened position in the world perhaps lay in my knowledge that I could never attain it. Or maybe I always knew that, for me, such a way of operating would be inconsistent with who I was and where my strengths lay. But the mere fact that the question existed for so long in me speaks to the power this brand of American masculinity exerts. And to this day, when confronted with such machoism, I have to remind myself to neither back down, nor push back, but to simply exist alongside it.

I turn off the television and notice a sign on the wall I failed to see when Shawn first showed me around. By the clothes rail in the back of the room beside the sink it reads, "Do not use towels for cleaning boots, guns, or blood. Old rags have been provided for this purpose." I scan the room, but no such rags are in evidence. Luckily, I'm wearing Nikes. Nor have I shot anyone, so consequently there is no blood.

And there's another sign. This one is located beside the old mini fridge, plunked on top of the dresser. "No cleaning or storing fish in rooms. They must be kept in your own cooler, no exceptions." As we're deep in the desert with no water for miles, I would agree that this makes good sense, since any fish are bound not to be the freshest.

I peel the brown-and-orange bedspread off and toss it in the corner. While Shawn has, I hope, changed the sheets since the last visitor, it's unlikely that the polyester spread has seen a wash in…

Once the lights are out, I sigh heavily, relieved to be in bed after a long day. Then I hear it—breathing, deep, hoarse, and rhythmic. Perhaps it's Carl in room 3. I snap on the lights. Naked, I rise and put my ear to the wall. No sound comes from next door. The breathing is coming from inside my room. I whirl around, I look under the bed, I get very still in the night. The breathing persists, slow and labored. After a long time, I zero in on it. The Darth Vader impersonation is coming from the ancient mini fridge. There are no fish, nor anything else inside, so I unplug it. The room is instantly silent.

Relieved, I fall quickly to sleep. Two hours later I'm woken by what sounds like shattering glass. I listen in the dark, decide it's nothing, and try to fall back to sleep.

A half hour later, just as I'm drifting back off, another noise like shattering glass startles me. I sit bolt upright in bed. On goes the light, and I stalk the room once again. "The fridge!" I exclaim at last. Since I unplugged it, the ice that had long formed on the tiny freezer must have dislodged and crashed to the bottom. I open the door and water pours all over my feet. I grab one of the towels I didn't use to clean my nonexistent gun and dry my legs.

Before I can get the light off again, the Seisco water pump on the back wall beside where the old rags aren't starts knocking and shuttering. Carl must have gotten up to use the toilet next door. I go back to bed. An hour later I'm woken by the rattling and bucking sound again, then again an hour later. Carl must have prostate issues. At four thirty in the morning I'm woken for the last time.

Since it's ninety miles to the first food and I'm already hungry, I decide to bathe and hit the road. The showerhead is mounted on the wall not far below my shoulders. I'm not sure why old plumbing was done this way, but I read somewhere that it was to preserve women's beehive hairdos in the 1960s. This makes as much sense as anything at this point.

A few kittens skitter away as I slip my room key through the mail slot of the locked office door. Disappointed not to say goodbye to Shawn, I'm on the road at first light.

Marfa, Texas

The sun rises in my rearview mirror as I head west out of Comstock on two-lane Route 90. The rolling hills give out when I reach the Stockton Plateau, and the vista stretches out into arid grasslands. Honey mesquite brush, as well as Vasey oak speckle the dirt. In Fort Stockton, I can finally get some breakfast at the Sagebrush Café.

I ask my middle-aged waitress how far it is to Wink.

"No idea."

"How long have you lived here?" I ask.

"My whole life."

The white-haired man at the next table tells me it's sixty miles. "You in the oil business?" he goes on. "There's no other reason to go to Wink."

"Going to the Roy Orbison Museum," I tell him.

He looks at me a long time, nonplussed. "Huh," he says at last. "Learn somethin' new every day."

The loneliest man in rock 'n roll spent his lonely teenage years in Wink, Texas. It informed a lot of who he became. Elvis Presley said that Orbison had "the most perfect voice" and called him "the greatest singer in the world."

For some reason I've never really examined, I've always felt an affinity for Roy Orbison. And while "pilgrimage" is perhaps too strong a word, I'm close enough to consider the museum sort of on my way.

The already stark land above Fort Stockton has been ravaged by the extraction of oil and natural gas. Eternal flames burn eerie atop flare stacks near and distant. Large trucks raise dust on dirt roads. Unused and discarded machinery corrodes in disorganized clusters. Litter blows across the landscape.

I bounce over the train track and enter Wink, population 882—and declining. Not far along Hendricks Boulevard is a small, whitewashed storefront between a vacant lot and a boarded-up brick building. The word "MUSEUM" has been hand-painted in block letters over the door. The wind is blowing hard when I approach the piece of paper taped to the glass. Three names and numbers are listed, instructing me to call and someone will come down and open the museum. I call them all. Only Barbara answers. She's out of town today.

"Nooo!" I plead. "I've driven hours."

"I'll be happy to show you anytime tomorrow," Barbara tells me.

Defeated, I sit on the bench out front and stare across the street to Curley's Grocery (closed down) and the empty lot beside it. A plastic bag caught in the branches of a dead tree blows uselessly, while trucks hauling sand under tarps being lifted by the wind rumble by and choke the street with dust.

I'm not sure why I've become fixated on seeing this place. I didn't even know the museum existed until a few days earlier, when I saw it in small letters in the corner of my map. And maybe that's why I've been singing Roy's classic, "Blue Bayou," in my head for the past several days. Whatever the reason, I feel an outsized despondency.

Or maybe I do know why I'm so disappointed.

A study by KFF (formerly known as the Kaiser Family Foundation) reports that twenty-two percent of men say they "often or always feel lonely."[1] The US Surgeon General has declared "an epidemic of loneliness and isolation."[2] Japan, along with the United Kingdom, has appointed a "Minister of Loneliness,"[3] while the World Health Organization has launched a Commission of Social Connection to combat the problem.[4] Even America's favorite cuddly sex therapist, Dr. Ruth, in her later years, talked less about sex and more about loneliness. And I seem to be encountering a great deal of it on the road lately.

Maybe the man who gave us "Only the Lonely," "One of the Lonely Ones," "Loneliness," and so many more has some answers for me.

I call Barbara back and set a time for tomorrow.

But I can't stay here.

Two hours southwest is the trendiest town in West Texas. Marfa. Artist Donald Judd came here in the 1970s and began what has grown into a creative oasis of sorts. Walking around town, poking my head into various hipster spaces and galleries, I'm reminded of Marcel Duchamp's line, "It's art if I say so." I'm sure this speaks only to my own limited sensibility, but I don't have the time of day for most of what I see in the sleek galleries or reclaimed gas stations. I'm much more interested in the Hotel Presidio.

It was here that Elizabeth Taylor, Rock Hudson, and, especially compelling to me, James Dean stayed while filming *Giant*, Dean's third and final film before his premature death at twenty-four. In his lightning flash of a career, Dean set the bar for depicting lonely, alienated youth that has never been approached.

The hotel is filled with memorabilia and behind-the-scenes photographs of the filming. One such photo is of Dean and Liz Taylor messing around on set in the desert. I snap a shot of the picture and for no reason that I can think of send it to Matthew. Within minutes he sends me one in return. It's an image of a smiling Dean behind the wheel of the Porsche Spider that would take his life in a high-speed crash a few days later. And now I realize why I sent him that photo. Thirty years earlier that picture of Dean in the car sat on top of the television in the Hollywood Hills bungalow that Matthew and I briefly shared.

I try to check in to Dean's old room, 223, but it's booked out.

"It usually is," Kelly, the heavily tattooed desk clerk, informs me. Turns out I'm not the only one looking for some solidarity with a ghost.

It's then in the lobby that I fall into conversation with a man in his early forties. He's square and solidly built with close-cropped hair and a long, almost ZZ Top–style beard. This is Aaron. Aaron is an air force veteran, former roughneck on an offshore oil rig, and current EMT. He's just come from Bible study in nearby Fort Davis.

Aaron recently moved to Marfa from Cat Springs, eight hours to the south and east, near Houston. He isn't so sure about his new neighbors. "We came down here for my wife's job, but I'll tell you something, most of the guys here need a good ass whoopin'. None of 'em have calluses on their hands."

I mention that this might not be the most charitable attitude for a man who's just come from Bible study.

"I follow God's rules, not man's," Aaron says.

I'm not sure what to do with that, so I let it pass. I ask if he's formed any new friendships here in town.

He considers briefly, then shakes his sturdy head. "Maybe one."

Aaron is wary and seems more comfortable with silence, something I've encountered with a certain type of man on this road trip. I just sit and nod my head.

"But I got three 'get in the truck' friends back home," Aaron starts up again.

"Get in the truck?"

"Yeah. Johnny, Leonard, and Reuter. Uncle Johnny, I don't see him much now, once every couple years, but if I call him and say, 'Hey, fucker, come get me,' he'll get in the truck and drive the nine hours, no questions asked. I trust him as much as I trust myself. He knows everything. One hundred percent." Aaron pauses and considers. "And if there's a disturbance in the Force—"

"The Force?"

"Like *Star Wars*," he says. "We can feel it. We haven't talked in months, but I'll call him up 'cause I feel something, and I'll say, 'What's wrong?' And he'll say 'Nothing,' but I'll know it's bullshit. 'What's wrong?' I'll ask again, and we'll talk about it. We're apart, but are we really apart? I just know I have a good friend."

Once Aaron loosens up, he has a lot to say on the topic.

"Leonard and Reuter too. Sometimes we're in a situation, maybe it goes sideways, we don't even talk to each other, but we don't have to. We just do what needs to be done. We're like dogs. We just know. They have that sense. Whatever that bond is, we have it."

Aaron's tone is softer now, and he sounds almost surprised when he says, "When I talk to them, I get me." The tender admission strikes me, particularly from a man who peppers his conversation with tough guy phrases like, "I don't start things, but I finish them."

"Look"—Aaron snaps his edge back into place—"I don't show emotion. I'm not good at it. But these guys, they've seen more emotion from me than my wife. I pour stuff out and they reciprocate. I'm not gonna be judged. There's no judgment."

I nod. Then Aaron feels the need to qualify his disclosure. "Don't get me wrong. We knock each other down, in a manly way. 'Quit crying like a baby,' that sort of thing. It's an abusive loving relationship." He laughs. "The more abusive the better." He laughs louder. Then he settles. "But they're the only guys I've ever said 'I love you' to."

That admission hangs between us.

"They're older," Aaron says finally, "particularly Uncle Johnny…I don't want to know when that day comes…I'll be alone…That'll be different."

Since Aaron is hinting at a loneliness much on my mind here in West Texas, I ask if he's ever lonely.

"Never," he snaps, dismissing the thought instantly. I'll take Aaron at his word, but experience tells me that when someone answers as fast and sharp as Aaron just did, it's a topic that frightens them.

Wink, Texas

A cold, early-morning wind is blowing through Marfa. I'm standing on the corner of South Highland Avenue and East Waco Street, hunched over a breakfast burrito, making an internal calculation. Do I drive the two-plus hours back through a heartless expanse to Wink, as I arranged with Barbara, or continue on toward El Paso, up into New Mexico and across Arizona and Nevada to Northern California toward my meet-up with Don? It's a long grind, and the rule of the road is simple—never go back.

But sometimes—as my friend John told me while we were camping on the Green River—"Rules are for fools."

"Fuck it." And I toss the remains of my breakfast into a nearby dumpster.

There are sections of the nearly 200,000 square miles of the Chihuahuan Desert, like the area just outside Marfa, that contain dramatic and changing vistas, mesas and buttes with sheer cliffs. But the vast majority of it does not. Creosote bush dominates the land for miles, hours. It's broken only with occasional yucca and agave. It's desperate land. And it's easy to grow unsettled, frightened even, in the endless expanse.

This feeling is not helped by the audiobook I'm listening to, Joseph Conrad's *Heart of Darkness*. Much of Conrad's descriptive genius in depicting the Congo River and the jungle of West Africa might easily apply to the desert of West Texas—"This stillness of life did not in the least resemble a peace. It was a stillness of an implacable force brooding over an inscrutable intention. It looked at you with a vengeful aspect." There's an ever-present knowing that the desert is only allowing me safe passage at its pleasure, which, with a flat tire or a blown gasket, might be rescinded at any moment. Like Conrad's narrator, I feel like I'm moving through "something great and invincible, like evil or the truth," that the land is merely "waiting patiently for the passing away of this fantastic invasion." This desert is not my friend. I try to call Seve, but my phone has no reception.

Then, beyond charmless Pecos, I'm back in the scarred crust of oil country. And when I bump over the railroad track, I'm in Wink again.

The wind is still blowing, and Barbara is waiting for me. She's white-haired, chatty, and "So happy this worked out. We get about ten, maybe fifteen visitors a month, and it breaks my heart when folks want to see our museum and we can't accommodate them."

The walls of the one-room shrine are lined with 45s, newspaper articles, posters for concerts. There are Roy's high school yearbooks. Under his 1957 senior picture, a shot of a sandy-haired boy with large glasses, is the quote,

> *To lead a western band*
> *is his afterschool wish,*
> *And of course, to marry*
> *A beautiful dish.*

"He tried out for the football team," Barbara tells me.
"How'd that work out?" I ask.

"Not so well. He was bullied a lot in school. That's why he went to Suzie Grey. She was a hairdresser who lived across the alley from Roy. Knocked on her door. He thought it would make him look tougher to have black hair."

Barbara's sincere affection for Roy, and the reverence on display in this small room, confirms the wisdom of retracing my steps through the desert—even before Barbara bends down behind the glass counter.

She comes up with something wrapped in a beige cloth. She places it gingerly atop the glass display case and slowly unwraps a cigar box–shaped container. Inside it are a pair of the glasses—Roy's iconic lavender-tinted lenses inside thick black frames. She handles them like the precious relic they are and holds them aloft. They catch the light.

"Can I try them on?" I almost whisper.

Barbara gasps. "Oh…" She looks around. There is no one else in the place (or anywhere in Wink, from what my two visits reveal). She considers.

I give her my best longing look.

"Okay," she says at last. "Maybe just for a minute."

The glasses are heavy and the thick lenses completely opaque. I can't make out anything through them at all. Roy was almost totally blind.

And it dawns on me that it was Roy's frailty that always attracted me to him, and that this frailty, quite the opposite of a liability, was his greatest asset, what he had to offer the world. Yet it makes sense growing up in rural Texas in the mid-twentieth century, a place filled with hard men like those I've recently met, that Roy felt the need to armor himself from the tip of his hair to his toes in black, and why he always wore sunglasses to shield himself.

For so long I hated my own feelings of vulnerability. But that frailty gave me so much—it fostered a sensitivity and perceptiveness that in time grew into my greatest strengths.

I imagine I can understand a fraction of how much it cost Roy to transmute the pain and loneliness he felt into something communal and shared. Confessing, "I'm so tired of feeling lonely, I still have some love to give" in his tremulous and soaring voice, it allowed the rest of us to admit to our own pain and yearning, to feel seen, less alone, maybe even to feel understood. His music created something quite the opposite of his trademark loneliness—it created connection. And the ghost of it is still on the wind in lonely West Texas.

John

Sandia Park, New Mexico

I should see the skyline of El Paso ahead, but the wind has kicked up such dust and sand that there's nothing visible through the golden-brown haze. I peel north along Route 54 and finally leave Texas behind.

Coming up from the south, the first thing of any substance that a traveler comes to in New Mexico is an area of white nothing. It was in this isolated corner of the desert that the first atomic bomb was set off on July 16, 1945, in a spot dubbed the Trinity Site, in a place called the White Sands Missile Range. In an odd logistical maneuver, White Sands National Park lies entirely within this still active missile range. And a long walk over its towering, undulating gypsum sand dunes in the howling wind leaves me feeling sandblasted and scrubbed clean. White Sands is the kind of thrilling and unexpected discovery that makes a traveler grateful to have left home.

Just to the north, while I'm cutting through the Mescalero Apache Reservation, my phone rings. Matthew is out walking his dog and has news regarding his scheme to get rich quick buying foreign currency that we discussed back in Lexington.

"Sport, you need to buy some Venezuelan bolivar," he tells me with urgency.

"What? Why?"

"Do you want to be rich or not? Just do what I'm telling you."

"What about those Vietnamese dong I bought?"

"The dong are going to come in, but the bolivar are going to happen first."

"Who told you this?"

"My person. Don't worry about it. We're gonna get the call very soon. Maybe tomorrow. Just get the bolivar."

"Really?"

"Yeah, we're going to get an 800 number. We'll call that and set up a time to go get our money from one of several banks."

"The dong or the Venezuelan thing?"

"Are you listening? The bolivar. It's going first, but it could be both. Just be ready."

"And you really think this is going to happen?" Matthew can hear the doubt in my voice.

"Hey, Mr. Cynic, just be ready."

I assure my friend that I am.

The following morning the wind is still up and heading north through central New Mexico on US Route 285, strong gusts buffeting the car. Something ahead rolls across the two-lane road—tumbles, actually. Getting closer, I see that it's Russian thistle, that invasive, noxious nuisance and iconic character of the American West—aka tumbleweed.

"Wow, cool!" I say aloud to the empty car, exposing my East Coast urban roots.

I'm headed deep into the desert for a night of "retreat."

On nearly every stop along the way of this cross-country improvisation, I've simply rolled into town and selected a place to sleep. But last night, after finding more than several large and unwholesome-looking spiders in the bed of my downtrodden motel, I tumbled down an internet rabbit hole and came upon a private retreat center in the middle of the desert somewhere between Albuquerque and Santa Fe. What makes it particularly appealing to someone like me—it serves just one guest at a time.

Then, in a trick of the mind that follows its own dictates, my friend Bellamy comes into my thoughts. Perhaps because he was among the first to point out to me something that anyone with eyes could see (except apparently, me), that I was decidedly not a "joiner."

We met in June of 1992. I was played out. A hopeless drunk at twenty-nine, a round-the-clock drinker, I checked in to the detox unit of a hospital on West Fifty-Ninth Street in New York City. For a week I did the Librium shuffle and shared a room with a tender, crossdressing junkie who was in on vacation, taking a break from life on the street and desiring nothing more than "three hots and a cot."

Bellamy was the head counselor on the unit. He had a wild intellect, a rock 'n roll past, and renegade notions about alcohol abuse and sobriety. He was neurotic, obsessive, gentle, and curious about who I was beyond the mess I was in. After I got myself cleaned up, we stayed in touch. Bellamy was the first and most important friend I made in my early sobriety.

As my drinking had grown worse—and both Seve and Eddie had moved away, leaving a large cavity—I'd pulled away from others and was hanging out only with other drinkers in dark neighborhood dives. I felt as alone as I ever had.

Once I dried out, I had to learn, to a very real degree, how to interact without alcohol. Bellamy was patient and supportive, and his faith in me allowed me to begin believing in myself as well.

We talked nightly on the phone, often for hours at a time. Bellamy was an academic. I was decidedly not. He was an atheist. I believed in something—although I would have been hard-pressed to tell you what that was. (I wouldn't be much better at telling you today.) He had fluid and questioning views on sobriety, while I was more pragmatic. We became dear friends, and I trusted him utterly.

In time, life filled in for us both. We spoke and saw each other less frequently, but I remained close with "wordy Bell" as my wife affectionately called my loquacious friend. After years and years of sobriety, Bellamy decided to drink again, using phrases like "harm reduction" to justify what sounded to me like nonsense. I couldn't get used to my friend with a glass of red wine in his hand.

Bellamy's experiment didn't work out well, and he diminished. We slipped away from each other. I saw little of him during the final decade of his life. The last time we spoke, I impulsively called Bellamy from the street—he seemed confused, talking with grandiloquence of trivial things. I missed my friend, but my friend was in many ways already gone. When his son eventually called to tell me Bellamy had died, I wasn't surprised. Six months later his ex-wife invited me to a celebration of life for Bellamy. I of course agreed to attend, but on the day of the gathering something came up and I didn't go.

I was shocked by my action. I still am. I haven't forgiven myself for not showing up—perhaps I'll need to forgive my friend his human frailty first.

Turning off the pavement, my rental Chevy Malibu bounces over a washboard dirt road. Five miles down the deteriorating track, thoughts of Bellamy and my failings are replaced by a more immediate concern—the sudden loud rattle under my hood. Will my Hertz insurance cover me when the imminent breakdown finally happens? I stop to open a cattle gate, and the car shudders on toward a small, elegant cabin on a platform below a low cliff set amid juniper and yucca.

Raymond, mid-forties, athletic, with sandy hair, is the host for my one-day retreat. He wastes no time on small talk, asking why I'm there and what I'm hoping to achieve in my brief time. I want to confess that I'm just looking for a clean bed and a good night's sleep, but under the intensity of Raymond's probing gaze, I'm suddenly spilling the goods on reclaiming my friendships and about talking with men across America on the topic, learning what I can.

It turns out that Raymond has long been pondering the same question of male friendship, and he's eager to compare notes. He immediately sets us off on a hike into the desert that I didn't request him to lead me on—then starts right in on how men and women handle their friendships differently.

"Women," he begins, "have more of an intuitive sense that friendship is not optional. They know they need their tribe. And stereotypically, women are more emotionally inclined and available. If a man has a problem, often, instead of seeking out a buddy to go have a beer or go fishing, he'll not look for help or tell anyone. It's just more instinctive for women to seek help."

I mention Carl, who I met at the motel in West Texas, who was out riding his motorcycle alone, contemplating a big decision in his life. "But I wonder if it isn't a bit like that Abraham Lincoln quote, 'The man who has himself for a lawyer has a fool for a client.'"

Raymond nods. "It's our Achilles. The superhero. He takes action. Figures it out on his own, doesn't complain."

I'm finding Raymond a strange mix—he's being generous with himself and has clearly spent time contemplating what it means to be a man in the world today. He sees the value in doing so and demonstrates an appetite for the topic. Yet I find it difficult to relax fully into our conversation. It feels as though Raymond is constantly assessing me, monitoring. Is it a whiff of insecurity I'm picking up on, of classic male defensiveness when broaching the topics of feelings and sensitivity? The effect is that it reads as slightly combative—and it's something I experience often with men, something I've been guilty of myself. Maybe like the rest of us, Raymond's simply been hurt in the past and has developed a protective shell, a mask—as Dale back in Tupelo labeled it.

Then, without prompting, Raymond takes up the theme that's been circling since I hit the desert back in Texas. "I think everyone is lonely, particularly men. So few have any encouragement or any direction. We're in a place in history where we live in a hyper-individualist, separated culture. We don't need a clan for survival anymore. And men spend far less time together than we used to. But the psychological effects are apparent."

When I spout some of my recently learned statistics on the adverse health effects of loneliness, Raymond appears to eye me with slightly more regard.

I laugh silently and am reminded of my daughter, Willow. She once told me that by simply stating a statistic, even a false one, you appear vastly more knowledgeable and command more respect. I make a mental note to text her my findings.

"But don't get me wrong," Raymond says. "I don't think men a hundred, two hundred, five hundred years ago were sitting around all day talking about their feelings. I don't romanticize it.

"Life was just so damn hard, they needed each other. If you weren't part of a community, a tribe, everything was harder.

Togetherness was more of a necessity. But"—Raymond lifts his finger for emphasis—"the point is, you had support. You weren't alone. You didn't have to figure out every damn thing yourself. And it's better for us to be together than apart. We're pack animals. It feels good when you feel a part of something, when you're watching out for someone and they're watching out for you."

The wind kicks up, and we take shelter behind large overhanging bedrock, surrounded by cholla cactus. Raymond, simultaneously reticent and impassioned, is just getting warmed up. "You watch *Band of Brothers*—it's the rare guy who finishes watching that and doesn't feel there's not something missing in their life. Or *I Heart Huckabees*. The bond that Mark Wahlberg has with Jason Schwartzman is one that every guy longs for, for someone who knows you're there, someone who gives a damn."

I consider confessing that I never saw either, but Raymond appears almost on the verge of tears discussing this—a nerve has been exposed.

"Mmm." I nod, aiming for neutrality. Then, feeling Raymond needs more from me, I ask, "Do you have that kind of connection in your life?"

"Not as much as I'd like." He talks about his experience with nationwide men's organizations like the Art of Manhood and Illumen, and their "rites of passage" and "initiator" programs.

I confess my resistance to such orchestrated, monetized efforts at masculine intimacy.

"It's quality stuff," Raymond assures me. "For someone to call out your goodness, that can be profound."

"I bet," I say, "but there's also the whole topic of organized men's groups being controversial. How some have come under fire for nurturing misogynistic ideas."

Raymond nods.

I keep going. "And there's the charge of creating a climate that allows for the whole 'incel' ideology to flourish, which has of course been linked to violence against women."

Raymond sits with this for a moment. "I know they're out there. But in my experience of healthy men's groups and literature, the message is always that you need to do *your* work so you don't manifest these traits and whatever other negative propensities that might arise from one's imperfect upbringing. And that it's actually the men who refuse to consort with men, be honest with their pain and wounding, and commit to a healing path that become the misogynists."

The wind blows through the arroyo.

In an effort to create those kinds of healthy experiences closer to home, Raymond has organized his own men's groups, with minimal success. "I'm a loyal friend, always initiating, following up, but I found I was the one doing the vast majority of the work. Eventually if things aren't reciprocal, you just let them go. And building that tribe from nothing, it's difficult. The most powerful thing I learned is that in the deepest bonds there's a founding experience that brings people together. Some metaphorical, or even literal enemy they're facing together, or some project they're doing or quest they're after, and that creates a bond much deeper than having coffee or asking someone 'what's the state of your emotional life?' It's more of a doing."

There's a very real yearning in Raymond, and I wonder why, if he feels such a pull toward fellowship, he's chosen to isolate himself, his wife, and his teenage daughter. I risk asking if it's an assertion of ego that's fueling an idea of something grand out here in the lonely

New Mexican desert. Raymond is silent a long time. His answer, when it comes, treads around the edges of my question.

"We came out here with a missionary mindset. To help people, to facilitate whatever it is they come out here to the retreat to process. It's rewarding work." He looks off, suddenly appearing exhausted. "But yeah, I'm kind of a one-man band." He considers some more. "It's a sacrifice, but…"

Clouds above pass quickly over the sun, casting and recasting the desert in clarity and shadow. I could be wrong, but I sense in Raymond a man holding fast to a dream he's not sure he believes in anymore.

It can be difficult to course-correct. It can appear as a tacit admission of defeat, or failure, or of being wrong, qualities that—especially for men—can be equated with weakness. And weakness, as I've seen on this trip, can be perceived as the most unmanly of traits. I'm tempted to share some of this thinking with Raymond. If we were friends, I'd like to think I'd take the chance. I also want to lighten his mood, suggest he move back to town, maybe join a basketball league. But I don't want him to think I'm making light of his commitment.

Back in my well-considered cabin, I switch on the flames in the automatic fireplace and pace around. I can't settle. I've still got a lot of country to cross.

So I leave.

When I tell Raymond I'm going, he nods in slow and considered understanding. Walking me to my car, he assures me that I'm "on a noble quest."

"I'm not so sure about that." I shrug, and reach for the door handle. "I just want to see my friends."

Bouncing away on the red-dirt road, my eyes go to the rearview mirror. Raymond has already turned away and, with his head lowered, is trudging back up the hill. I round a bend and he's gone.

It's not so much that I didn't want to stay at Raymond's retreat. It's that I want to be somewhere else... and that somewhere is standing on a corner in Winslow, Arizona.

It's nearly impossible to get from Albuquerque, New Mexico, to Winslow, Arizona, other than on Interstate 40. So I head due west surrounded by eighteen-wheel trucks rumbling across America—maybe it's the desert air, but they jangle my nerves less than usual. The interstate here supplanted famous Route 66, and as I approach the Continental Divide east of Gallup, sheer cliffs appear to have popped directly up from the flat earth like those Whac-A-Mole games. I begin to recognize this red-rock landscape. And while I've never been here before, I do have kids. And when they were little, my kids watched the Pixar movie *Cars*. A lot. The film about talking autos was set in this desert landscape, along the ghost of Route 66. The precise animation and repeated viewings have embedded this alien land deep into my psyche and given me a sense of history with a place I've never known in a way that only the movies can do. Nostalgic flashes of my children in their early youth cause me to laugh. Then a large truck shifts lanes to pass a larger truck and almost runs me off the road.

There's not much to Winslow except the corner of Kinsley and Second Street. There's not really much to the corner of Kinsley and Second Street either, except that it's where the city council decided to place a sign commemorating the Eagles' iconic song

"Take It Easy" and erected a statue of Jackson Browne and one of Glenn Frey, who co-wrote the hit. They've even parked a flatbed Ford on the corner ("It's a girl, my Lord/in a flatbed Ford...").

I take a half dozen selfies standing on the corner. Then, sitting on a bench (on the corner) while the nearby trinket shop pipes Eagles hits out into the air—as it does all day, every day—I text a photo to Matthew. This is precisely the kind of stupidity he can appreciate.

OMFG! comes the reply in short order.

I send one to Eddie.

A pair of excited boomers arrive and snap selfies, exactly as I just did. And then another pair. Winslow is making the most of its claim to fame.

My phone pings. *Awesome!!* Then, *Go to La Posada.*

The other attraction in sleepy, isolated Winslow is La Posada Hotel, and had Eddie not mentioned it I would have missed it.

The best hotels, regardless of their degree of luxury, create the sense that they've been preparing for your arrival for a long time. Opened in 1930, La Posada was the brainchild of Fred Harvey, who is credited with "civilizing the west" with hotels strung along the Santa Fe Railway. Albert Einstein, Amelia Earhart, Clark Gable—all took the train deep into the desert to stay at this sprawling hacienda.

It's still easy to feel the relief early travelers must have experienced when coming upon such a soft landing amid such harsh terrain. The south entrance to the hotel lies directly on the tracks. I sit in a wicker chair on the veranda beside the wishing well for a long while, watching trains couple and uncouple, arrive and depart. This (un)activity is surprisingly engaging in the otherwise still air. The illusion of movement created gives a weary traveler a sense of continued propulsion while doing absolutely nothing. I imagine Seve sitting beside me—it was his example that taught me to appreciate such mundane pleasures.

I scroll through my phone looking at all the texts I've sent back and forth with Seve, Matthew, and Eddie since we reconnected. Alone in Winslow, I feel surrounded by friendship.

The following morning, on the way out of town I need to fill my tank. My hand squeezing the handle, I can feel gas rushing through the hose. A black bird darts past me. Rarely do I feel this present, this at home in myself. And it strikes me that the comfort of my male friends' support manifests in me so differently from the support of my wife. Their support is not better, not more complete, but it lands differently in me, relieves something different.

So often I'm preoccupied with the worries of the day, or with perpetually overriding concerns—providing for my family, ensuring my kids' futures, seeing after the care of my ailing mother. I squarely feel the burden of responsibility. I am the one who has to ensure that everyone is safe, has a home, is provided for and happy.

Is this just old-school male indoctrination and sexism? The fact that my wife is generally much more capable than I am, or that no one keeps their head in a crisis better than Dolores, does little to dispel this (delusional?) sensation.

Regardless, the pressure of my (mis)perception presses down and creates a weight I habitually carry. It is a dominant experience in my life, and something my male friends can identify with and understand with nothing more complex than a shrug of "of course."

Sedona, Arizona

I'd been to Sedona years earlier and recall it as both splendid and silly. Physically majestic, surrounded by red-rock buttes and forests of pine, with clean air under a thin blue sky, Sedona has instant curb appeal. It also has, by my unofficial reckoning, the most psychics, shops selling crystals, as well as aura-balancing salons in the country. A few hours southwest of Winslow, it's worth the slight swerve as I make my way toward the coast.

Neither a hater nor a searcher of that particular variety, I find myself simultaneously curious and bored by the commerce I find on Main Street. I wander in and out of the Heart Light Healing Center and the Crystal Vortex shop as well as the Mystical Bazaar—where I discuss getting my aura photographed. At Spiritstone Coffee on bustling Sacajawea Square in the heart of Uptown—the epicenter (vortex?) of New Age life in Sedona—I take a seat on a bench, looking out to the red-rock cliffs that preside over town, and fall into conversation with a wiry, blond man in his thirties.

Tim, who writes for the local newspaper, is interested in my road trip, and when I mention my morning insight at the gas station in Winslow—how men and women fill different emotional needs—my cross-country conversation continues.

"I'd ascribe what you're saying to the way our society segregates the experiences of men and women. It's taken for granted that men and women are inherently different, and that precludes the possibility of true communication with one another. Men are from Mars, women are from Venus, as that book says, yet there's no evidence to support that, in anthropology or sociology. What we come up with as far as gender roles is entirely a cultural construct that has nothing inherent about it. Societies change all the time, always have, always will. We're currently experiencing a transition in relation to gender identity."

While not certain I agree with all that, I express my gratitude to Tim for jumping in so wholeheartedly to discuss the topic with a stranger. He shrugs. "People are reluctant to discuss friendship because it has no immediacy, no monetary value, it won't further their careers."

I suggest that might be a bit cynical and tell Tim that my unscientific experience on the road has shown that once the surface is scratched, people have a lot of thoughts on the matter and have been eager to share them.

"I'm glad to hear that, and a little surprised. But look, social interaction releases dopamine and oxytocin, which have benefits to cognition, creativity, you name it. To a certain extent, the more people we have in our life, the better off we are. You get the feeling that you're not alone, which is wonderfully stabilizing. And working hand in hand with that is the knowledge that you're providing the same for someone else. It's reciprocal, it's balanced. It's our feelings of vulnerability that prompt us to seek out company and interaction with others."

"Vulnerability can be a four-letter word for men," I say.

Tim looks off toward the cliffs presiding over town. "Women are encouraged to build those interrelationships more than men, whereas men are encouraged to compete against each other. Men accomplish and move on."

Something in the simplicity and directness of this remark catches me up short. In the dozens of conversations I've had on the topic since leaving home, I haven't heard it put so succinctly. In my own experience, I've known that to be true in numerous instances. Life has been about achieving, with the majority of my friendships centering around work. When those work goals have been realized, the relationships, even those that have gone beyond shop talk and delved into more intimate terrain, have tended to fade.

We sip our coffees. My eyes follow two trim women in Lululemon gear walking left to right. Tim's gaze tracks two broad-shouldered men crossing right to left. We laugh. And something occurs to me.

"I had a friend who once said, 'I'd give most women I meet a spin at least once.' However crass that statement may be—and I'm making a broad generalization here—I think the majority of guys I know would agree. They'd sleep with most of the women they meet at least once. And I'd say that most male/female friendships that remain completely platonic do so because of the woman's choice, much more so than the man's. Again, I'm generalizing, but how does it work in the gay world?"

Tim's response comes easily, "The prospect of casual sex is an item on the friendship menu for men who are attracted to men." He considers for a moment, then continues. "Yes, in my experience, among those of us who are attracted to other men, it's pretty much a given. It doesn't have to be immediate, but you're always knowing that it could happen down the road.

"Case in point, a couple weekends ago I ended up in the shower with a couple friends of mine who I've known for about two years. That was the first time we'd done that. It had always kind of been on the table. It just hadn't happened. Then the opportunity was right." He shrugs. "It's always an option. That's just the attitude you have."

"From my experience," I say, "and from what I know of my other straight friends, hopping into the shower like that would alter the nature of the friendship. Is that your experience?"

"Not at all. And see, that's the thing—and I've had the conversation with other gay friends before—there is a level of casual comfort with easily available sex that does not readily transfer over into male/female interaction in society.

"There's also another angle of this to consider," Tim continues. "A lot of friendships begin with a casual hookup, and then you realize, 'Oh, we have other things in common and we can go from there.'"

"That does happen among heterosexuals as well."

"True."

Clouds slide across the sun. The air cools. Tim finishes his coffee and stands to head back to work.

"I'm glad you're doing this trip," he says. "True friends aren't often or easily found, and you want to hold on to them. It's worth the effort to travel to reconnect with them."

All of this active focus on the value of connection and reconnection is obviously having some effect on me—or maybe it's the Sedona vortexes—because I find myself reaching out to a man I met here just once, years ago. It's the kind of thing I would normally never consider if I were passing through town. Yet in short order, I'm sitting across the desk from Patrick Schweiss, an enthusiast in his fifties who runs the Sedona Film Festival. Posters of films I don't recognize adorn the walls of his office in a nearby strip mall.

"What are you doing here?" Patrick shouts by way of greeting, then shakes his head in bewilderment at hearing what I'm up to. Patrick is all smiles and admits to being, in his words, "compulsively social." "I know so many people, have so many acquaintances, I have guys I see all the time, whether it's golfing, going to the casino, going for a drink," and here he pauses, "but a true, deep male friendship?" He shakes his head. "That is a concept I can't really even grasp."

We laugh, and I appreciate his candor. Patrick is speaking easily for so many men who don't.

"I suppose I'm really missing out on something, but to tell you the truth, I've never even considered it." Patrick literally throws up his hands. "Male friends? I don't know if I'd even know how."

He smiles again and reaches for his phone. "But I do know who you need to talk with."

An hour later, just down the road beside the Global Center for Christ Consciousness (which describes itself as a New Age Spiritual Center, New Thought Church, and Energy Vortex), I meet up with Patrick's friend, a middle-aged man with a genial manner trying to get a small fire going in the enclosed yard beside the church. Derek leads a local men's group that meets weekly and ponders the question of what it is to be a man in today's world, and how to be a better one.

"There are about thirty of us. Usually about ten to twelve of us at a time gather here," Derek says, indicating the benches surrounding the firepit. He started the group in 2007, an outgrowth of his experience with the Mankind Project.

A global network of more than a thousand peer groups, the website for the Mankind Project boasts of its goals to create more responsible, emotionally mature, and spiritually aware men.

Derek took part in the group's signature Warrior Training Retreat, a forty-eight-hour experience that he says changed his life.

"It was a real rite of passage, the kind we don't get growing up in our society. There are a lot of fourteen-year-olds walking around in forty-year-old bodies."

"Why'd you join?" I ask. "What were you looking for?"

"I was always more comfortable with women. I'd never trusted men. I've never been a football guy or into the one-upmanship." Derek blows on the fledgling fire. "Men haven't been given permission to feel their feelings. A lot of men are walking around with a lot of wounds that have never been addressed. In our group we look at those unclaimed parts of ourselves. It's based in Jungian psychology and the work of Robert Bligh. Dealing with archetypes—the King, the Lover, etc. It's about being honest with yourself. What parts of my life aren't working?"

Phrases like "shadow work" and "accountability process" and "personal integrity" pepper Derek's description of the group's work.

His friend Joe, a tall, thin man with long hair under a brimmed hat, with a direct gaze and casually intense manner, joins us around the fire. "In this circle we create a safe container," Joe says. "The men have each other's back. The structure here creates friendship."

Derek leans in. "There are some things about the male experience that men feel more comfortable talking about with each other."

"This men's group is a safe place to share some of your deepest stuff. What you might not share with a woman." Joe, a landscaper by trade, waves away smoke from the shifting breeze. The wind chimes hanging from the corner of the church roof trill as evening comes on.

"It's about vulnerability," Derek agrees. "When you see a guy being super vulnerable, it gives you permission to be vulnerable as well. The bravest are the ones who are most vulnerable."

I think of Carl again, riding solitary through the West Texas desert on his motorcycle, and of John Wayne playing on my motel television. They may not agree.

"There's true strength in showing that vulnerability," Joe says. "Wrap it up in courage. Society has created a structure of what it is to be a man. A man can't be vulnerable or weak. Can't share his love for another man or he's gay. Derek and I have no problem sharing our love for each other. It's at the core of our relationship," Joe assures me, his gaze unwavering. "We're both straight men. Derek is my soul brother; I'd do anything for him."

Derek laughs. "Sometimes my wife says to me, 'You need to go to your men's group.'"

I'm reminded of Lew and Bobby, the retired cops I met back in Ohio. How Lew's wife will tell him he needs some "Bobby time."

"There's no doubt that any secure woman can see their man come back from a meeting empowered, lit up across the board," Joe enthuses. "And that's in everyone's best interest."

Derek laughs. "And sometimes it's a turn-on."

Joe remains serious. "Sure, that comes from deep sharing. Once you know yourself and can share yourself, that's sexy."

"So, why's it so difficult?" I ask.

"Shame," Derek says with matter-of-factness. "I'm gonna hide things about myself 'cause if you see too deep into me, you'll see what a piece of shit I really am. Therefore, I'm not gonna show you who I really am. As Freud said, 'Secrets make us sick.' You have secrets and you feel you won't be accepted. We deal with that toxic shame in our circle a lot.

"We'd both done a lot of work with groups, exercises where you're pushed to your limit, screaming, crying, and you get to your wound, and no therapy you've ever done can get you to that."

Before I can question that assertion, Joe clarifies, "Not that quick, anyway."

"It's a twenty-minute process," Derek says. "The 'carpet work' is very intense."

By "carpet work" Derek is referring to a literal carpet where the process takes place, a kind of emotional boxing ring. "It can be as simple as a man talking to different aspects of his personality by sitting in different chairs. 'My little boy says I need this…' 'My inner teenager says I want this…' Or it can be as literal as creating physical barriers for the man to burst through what's holding him back by finding his masculine intensity, literally breaking through physical restraints to reach something he wants or needs to feel complete."

Joe nods. "It's very structured. It all boils down to trust and love and being able to communicate that. Our goal is to take responsibility for ourselves, our feelings."

Joe's remark echoes what Raymond recently said to me in the arroyo, to "do *your* work."

We're quiet for a moment, the fire licking up into the purple sky. I confess that perhaps it's my defensiveness fostering the cynic in me, but I'm still quick to recoil at what I glibly call therapy games. I have a long distrust for such orchestrated insights.

Derek and Joe smile at me good-naturedly.

I can appreciate and respect the value these two (as well as Raymond and so many others) have found in such a process. And the bond between Derek and Joe is palpable and proof of the effectiveness of such emotional work. The three of us sit comfortably, watching the fire.

Derek speaks at last. "I can't tell you how many women have called me up and said, 'My husband doesn't have any friends. Can he join your group?'"

Monument Valley, Arizona

I retrace my steps north out of Sedona, regaining elevation and the Mogollon Rim. A quick and inexact glance at the map tells me I'm roughly halfway between Eddie in Cleburne, Texas, and Don in Oakland, California. I'm thinking I'll turn west at Flagstaff, a few miles up the road, and cut through Las Vegas for some quick fun, when Seve calls.

"Where are you now?" he shouts into the phone when I answer. I tell him.

"No kidding? Hey, do you remember that time when we were driving cross-country, and we met that guy who took us on a helicopter ride into the Grand Canyon?"

I flash on an image I hadn't thought of in thirty years—strapped into the front seat of a helicopter plunging down between canyon walls, hearing a panicked Seve in the seat behind me, shouting "Whooooa" through the scratchy headset.

"When we went over that rim, and the ground fell away"—Seve is laughing now—"man, my stomach just dropped."

"That helicopter scared the shit out of me," I say.

"How did we meet that guy?"

"No idea, probably in some bar. But I'll never do it again."

"You going to the canyon?"

"Wasn't planning to," and then right on cue a sign for US Route 180 and the Grand Canyon appears by the side of the road in front of me.

I take the exit. Vegas is out.

"I am now," I tell Seve. Lightning flashes on the horizon.

It of course makes no sense trying to describe to someone what it's like to stand at the rim of the Grand Canyon. Majestic, awe-inspiring, you've-never-seen-anything-like-it—words are insufficient. Statistics are equally unsatisfying—a mile deep, more than ten miles (at times nearly twenty miles) across, somewhere between five and seventy million years old, etc.

So I take a photo and send it to my wife, without a caption.

Where's that? she texts back.

The Grand Canyon, I type.

I watch my phone as the three dots blink for a moment. Then comes the reply.

Never heard of it.

My wife is often funnier than I expect her to be. And this constitutes our entire conversation regarding the big hole in the ground in northern Arizona that attracts about five million visitors a year.

I hike into the canyon along the switchbacks of Bright Angel Trail for a few hours and down through several millennia before retracing my steps. (Less than one percent of visitors go below the rim and down into the canyon that covers nearly two thousand square miles.) Walking has always clarified my thinking, and the input I've received from men of late has been circling, waiting to be sorted. *Perhaps it's all just simpler than I'm making it*, I conclude as I retake the rim of the canyon.

I spend the night in an old lodge at the edge of the ravine. More basic than La Posada in Winslow, it's likewise designed by Mary

Jane Colter and the brainchild of Fred Harvey. It retains a similar feel of the individual authenticity that went a long way in establishing how the American West would define itself, and still does.

Consulting my map before bed while trying to decide my route for the next day, my intent is to wrap around the canyon and head north for Page, Arizona. But while cross-referencing something on my phone, a photo of Monument Valley pops up.

I saw enough John Ford Westerns in those dark revival houses of Greenwich Village while skipping my college classes to instantly recognize the iconic and singular American landscape of sandstone buttes jutting up from the sprawling desert floor.

Page is out. Monument Valley is in.

My decisions are coming fast and loose now. And then my eye drifts up toward Wyoming on the map. My friend John lives in Wyoming. When all this began back at my kitchen table in New York, John was one of the men I called about getting together, but he was off mountain climbing in the Himalayas. He's usually gone on these types of trips for a few months. I have no idea when he's due back.

Like Don, John is a friend made in adulthood.

I decide to shoot him a text. *Dude, you still climbing?*

Quickly, a text comes back. *No. Back home, getting surgery on my shoulder tomorrow.*

I dial the phone.

"What the hell happened to you?" I say instead of hello.

"Dude!" John laughs. He's laughing as much at himself for calling me "Dude" as anything else. I'm fairly certain I'm the only person John—the well-brought-up son of a preacher—calls Dude. I take the blame for this, having called him Dude from the start. And as any guy will tell you, when one dude calls the other dude Dude, the second dude is all but obliged to reciprocate. And so, we are Dudes.

John fills me in quickly on his trip and his imminent shoulder surgery. I tell him I'm down at the Grand Canyon.

"Really? Listen, I'll be out of it for a few days," he says, "but then if you've got time, and if you're up for the drive, I'll be stuck here doing nothing. It would be great to hang out."

And just like that I've doubled my driving distance to the West Coast.

I quickly email Don to let him know it's going to take me a bit longer to make it to him.

The morning is cloudless and cold. US Route 64 is paved smooth, paid for with all those national park entrance fees. I track east through juniper and ponderosa pine, the road offering peekaboo views of the canyon for nearly thirty more miles—twice I come close to careening off the pavement as my head swivels. Fortunately, I'm impeded from going as fast as I'd like by a very slow-moving RV with the words "RENT ME" stenciled across its back.

Outside the park, the two-lane road turns rough and treeless desert begins to spread. An hour down the road I glance over at the passenger seat to where my road atlas of the fifty states always sits.

"Oh, shit!" It's not there.

I consider turning around. I call the hotel at the Grand Canyon. Housekeeping has not been to the room yet. We discuss them sending it to my home in New York. I drive on, glancing at the empty passenger seat. That map has become my companion, proof of my hard-earned miles, my touchstone for friendship. I make a U-turn.

Three hours later, map beside me on the passenger seat, I've returned to the exact same spot and make a right onto Route 160. It takes me onto the Navajo Trail and into the pastel hues of the Painted Desert. Needle grass dots the open prairie. Juniper and cliffrose top the mesas. The road is empty. The sky is vast. My mind drifts, and one cloud looks like a llama, another like Frosty the Snowman, a third like a pair of coupling aardvarks.

At the Navajo Welcome Center, I stop to buy an entrance ticket to Monument Valley (which sits on Navajo land), and as I walk back out through the door, I literally bump into a man in his mid-forties with a long black ponytail under a black Denver Broncos baseball cap, wearing a brown shirt with mother-of-pearl snaps and faded, dirty jeans and boots. Will is a member of the Navajo Nation and leads tours into the valley. We fall into easy conversation. A mix of edgy charm and guarded amiability, he's a complicated man to read.

"My grandmother eight generations back is from here," Will informs me. "Her name was Walks to the Water. This place is ground zero for me."

Will and his two brothers left for a time and went to work as welders on the Golden Gate Bridge, but all three felt the pull to return to what he calls the "four elements"—air, fire, water, and earth. He speaks of the oral tradition that was passed down to him and the legends he grew up hearing. "The history that you learned about us and our land was the European story. *His-story*, not *our* story." Walking back to his pickup, Will talks in detail about the energy in the earth, and with pride that the Spanish could never conquer Navajo land. "They couldn't find the water." He leans toward me. "It's in the rocks."

Will was raised in a hogan, a traditional Navajo dwelling constructed of three forked poles covered with sticks and mud, with his two brothers and four generations of women. "If someone was going to sneeze, I knew it five minutes before. We were close."

I ask if things are still the same.

Will leans against his truck. "The community is less strong. The older men still talk the tradition. It makes it interesting, but I've got other friends as well."

"Mostly Navajo?" I ask.

"American friends too. From New York, California." And his friends tend to be more men than women. "The conversation is different with men and women."

"In what way?"

"With men we're in the same boat. We tend to connect over work. We understand. Gotta bring it home." Distant thunder rumbles to the south, and Will absently turns his head in that direction.

"How many close male friends do you have?" I ask.

Will considers, then picks a number. "Thirty."

"Thirty?!" I exclaim. "How many would you call if your truck broke down a hundred miles away?"

"Any of them."

"I don't believe that," I say.

Will shows a slow grin. "But my granddaughter is my closest buddy. I call her Eskimo, because she was born during COVID and we couldn't kiss her, so we just rubbed noses."

"I don't think we call them Eskimos anymore," I say.

Will lets this pass. We stand looking out beyond the prickly pear and yucca toward East and West Mittens, the most iconic of the valley's famous buttes. The parking lot around us is nearly deserted. The wind has kicked up. Dark clouds are forming to the south. Will suggests I better get out to the valley's sixteen-mile dirt loop road before the rain arrives. "Take my number. If you get in any trouble out there, you give me a shout."

As we part, I call back across the parking lot. "What's the most important quality in those thirty close friendships?"

Will props an elbow on his truck, readjusts his cap, and calls back, "Being able to depend on each other."

Vernal, Utah

One of the more iconic images of the American West, the subject of countless photos, is that of a narrow two-lane track sweeping down and away, a long, straight line tapering to the base of the buttes of Monument Valley rising up from the distant desert under a vast blue sky. It's a thrilling vista, one capturing the rugged spirit of American individuality. But there's something in the image I've always found daunting as well—the lonely road, a solitary, potentially precarious journey ahead. As this trip has begun to show me, such isolation comes with a price.

Heading north out of the Navajo Nation along State Route 163 the day after my encounter with Will, those paradoxical feelings, possibility and perilous isolation, are strong in me when my eye goes to the rearview mirror.

I pull the car to the side of the road and get out to look back. Before me, or rather behind me, is the living image of the photo I've seen for decades—the road stretching down and away to a valley and the distant outcrops under an azure sky. I laugh. "There you are," I say out loud through the wind.

I cross the San Juan River at Mexican Hat, population 31, named for a nearby outcrop of rocks that looks like, well, a Mexican sombrero. When I turn north on US 191, distant showers are visible over the sandstone pinnacles of the Valley of the Gods to the west. Ninety miles up the road, I ease into Moab.

I was here once before, years earlier. Matthew was performing in a play at an unlikely theater in tiny Helper, a few hours north, and I'd come out to see him. Other than being the gateway to Arches and Canyonlands National Parks, Moab is known to be a mecca for mountain bikers. Matthew and I decided to go for a ride on his day off. My experience with off-road biking consisted of riding my three-speed over the curb as a child. Matthew was less skilled. At one of the many outdoor outfitters on Main Street I asked the young and athletic-looking man renting us bikes, "Where's the best place to go?"

"Slickrock Trail is probably the most famous route."

"Is it difficult?"

"Very."

"Like, do you think we could handle it?"

He looked me up and down.

"We're only here for one day," I said, trying to sound confident.

"Go for it," the young man said.

Matthew, who had gone outside for a cigarette, asked, "He give you an easy route?" as I came out.

"Yeah, we'll be fine," I said without meeting my friend's eye.

A few miles out of town in the desert we found an undulating, crevice-riddled, windblown sandstone expanse under a blistering summer sun. If it weren't for the white dashes painted on the aptly named slick rocks of the "trail," we would have had no idea where to attempt to go. After his third fall in less than twenty minutes (I only fell twice), Matthew called out, "I'm a Jew from Long Island. What the fuck am I doing out here!"

We kept the bikes—parked outside the nearest bar—for several more hours before returning them so as not to arouse suspicion from the athletic young man who'd rented them to us.

This time I'm not renting a bike, but I do text Matthew while eating tacos at Fiesta Mexicana on Main Street.

Don't ever remind me of that bike ride again, he texts back quickly.

You're lucky I still speak to you, comes a second text moments later.

In fact, lose my number, comes a third.

Sport! it was years ago! I text.

Who is this? comes the reply. *I don't recognize this number*

Because of the engine warning lights I'd been getting since Kentucky, I swapped out my rental car back in Dallas. But now, as I turn in for a quick look at Arches National Park, the engine warning light on this latest Chevy Malibu flares on as well. As I'm in the West, often traveling long distances over isolated roads, I don't want this anxiety hanging over me as it did down through Tennessee and Mississippi, then across Louisiana and half of Texas.

I reach for my phone. After long and looping negotiations with an automated operator, I am reduced to a screaming fit. "Speak to an agent. Speak to an agent! SPEAK TO AN AGENT!!!"

At last, a human comes on the line. The overly polite representative repeatedly puts me on hold. A Muzak version of "Up, Up and Away" fails to pacify me. Eventually I'm told that none of the agency's vaguely nearby rental outlets are interested in swapping out my car. But the company is willing to deliver one from Salt Lake City, and it should be to me in about eight hours.

I quickly weigh my options. "I'd rather deal with the possibility of breaking down," I tell the well-mannered representative.

"Entirely up to you, sir. We're happy to help."

Deciding to leave Arches for another day, I track the winding course of the Colorado River on twisting Route 128 through carved canyons of dramatic red rocks. The gorge is narrow and steep. Cottonwood and willow hug the snaking riverbank. Sandstone cliffs loom overhead. A lone golden eagle rides a thermal in a cloudless sky. American splendor.

In order to get due north, I'm forced to shimmy east on transcontinental I-70. A large black raven is perched atop the eighty-miles-per-hour speed limit sign when I cross into Colorado. Eventually I can turn north onto a lonely two-lane track. I pass three cars over the next seventy miles.

For the past few days, I've been listening to *Victory*, another Joseph Conrad novel, to accompany my drive, and a line jumps out at me. "A man drifts. It proves nothing, unless perhaps some hidden weakness of character."

In Dinosaur, Colorado, I make a left on Brontosaurus Boulevard and I'm back on US Route 40—the road on which I began this journey two thousand miles east in Atlantic City.

That I've so far driven more than triple those two thousand miles may give the appearance of my drifting across the country. Yet, while my character contains many weaknesses, drifting, despite my indirect route and occasional inner doubts, is not what has been happening over these miles. Something in revisiting, reclaiming, my friendships, is beginning to settle in me.

After crossing the border back into northeast Utah, I'm in the lobby of the Dinosaur Motel on Main Street in Vernal, looking for a vending machine to buy a bottle of water, when I hear a noise. I follow it to a cramped kitchen just off the lobby and come upon Darrell, the small, amiable man in glasses who checked me in a half hour earlier. He's in the process of cracking 220 eggs and placing them in Tupperware containers.

"Prepping breakfast for tomorrow," he explains. A recently retired schoolteacher, Darrell found himself working here because he was "looking for something to do. To get out of the house." Born in Salt Lake, raised in rural Washington, he's been in Vernal for a quarter century. Darrell is also an elder on the High Council of the Church of Jesus Christ of Latter-day Saints.

"Were you born into the Mormon Church?"

"My great-great-great grandfather was on his way out to the gold rush in California. He stopped off in Salt Lake on July 24, 1849, two years to the day after the pioneers settled. He liked what he saw and joined the church and never got to California."

I offer to help crack eggs, but Darrell has his rhythm.

"What exactly do you do on the High Council?"

"We have various responsibilities, supervise and coordinate the different wards. We advise." Darrell goes on like this in a general fashion that clarifies nothing to me.

A pickup truck rumbles by outside, its exhaust in need of attention.

"Are there women on the High Council?" I ask ignorantly.

Darrell shakes his head gently. "It's twelve men."

"You must be close with those men."

"Of course." Darrell cracks the last of the eggs and seals the final container, stacks it on top of two others and places them in the refrigerator. "But we're generally addressing church business.

I have to say that I find it easier talking with women. Maybe it's because I taught elementary school for twenty-five years, and most of the people I worked with were women."

I resist the urge to quote reports and statistics I've uncovered during my trip that speak to the issue Darrell is circling. I simply say, "A lot of men don't have male friends."

"I have some," Darrell equivocates, leaning now against the counter. "Some good friends, but we don't get together often."

When I press him on when the last time was, Darrell considers for a while and then can only shrug.

"Women tend to be more open," he goes on. "Men are more closed. It's difficult."

"Sometimes a common activity…" I suggest. "Ever into sports?"

"No, I never was, I played and taught piano. My family were musicians." He eases past me out of the claustrophobic kitchen and back into the lobby. Like a number of men I encounter on this trip, Darrell is both skittish to discuss the topic of male friendship and yet intrigued, not ready to let it go. "Like I say," Darrell picks up again just as I'm ready to let him get back to work, "I'm friends with the men doing church business, but going out to dinner just to get together…?" Darrell seems almost baffled by the idea.

"Yeah, women tend to cultivate their friendships more," I say.

"That's very true," Darrell exclaims, as if grasping a lifeline. "My wife goes out with her friends at least once a month. More."

"And with men," I start, almost hesitant to continue, "in certain circles, there can sometimes be a stigma about intimate male friendships, that there must then be a sexual component involved."

Darrell's voice goes quiet, almost to a whisper. "Well, I've heard of men going on those sort of trips... together... doing that sort of thing. I don't do that. I haven't ever thought about anything like that," Darrell assures me. "I only do that kind of thing with my wife."

Lander, Wyoming

It's eight a.m. and I'm in Betty's Diner, beside the local chapter of the Elks Club, a ten-minute walk along Main Street from the Dinosaur Motel. Men with bellies and beards and wide-hipped women fill the place. Large windows look out onto the passing traffic and across to the Ford dealership, its lot crammed with brand-new pickup trucks. A plate filled with biscuits and brimming with gravy is hurried by. A woman with tattoos down her arm is cutting pancakes for the small child beside her who wears a Spider-Man hat. "I'll have number three," a bald man looking at the laminated menu tells the waitress at the next table, then looks up to her and smiles. There's laughter in the room. I've witnessed variations on this scene across the nation. And if I come away from this cross-country odyssey with one conclusion, it is that breakfast in America is the most hopeful meal of the day.

Back in the car, crossing the Flaming Gorge Dam and Green River, heading north into Wyoming, the road climbs through aspen and pine. As always, I find myself growing anxious as I ascend through the mountain pass, only to feel expansive relief on the descent. The land grows dry and brown and beige, the views broaden. There is parched sage and yellow grass. Then I'm traveling for a long time over a high and exposed plateau, and across open range. Past Eden, population 245, I make an impulsive decision and turn onto State Route 28 toward Lander.

It would be odd if I didn't.

The road here is straighter for longer than any I've yet driven. The Wind River mountain range is to my left—I've spent time in those mountains. Crossing the Sweetwater River the road sweeps north and west, I skirt the edges of the Shoshone National Forest, and soon irrigated fields bring me back to a chapter in my past.

Growing up in suburban New Jersey, I went camping just once—during my brief and failed career as a Cub Scout. We got rained on and came home in the middle of the night, soaked and miserable. But in my early thirties I decided I needed to learn how to fend for myself in the great outdoors. I enrolled in a month-long course at the National Outdoor Leadership School (NOLS), based in Lander, Wyoming. I spent twenty-eight challenging days in the Absaroka Mountains with a dozen other students and three instructors. We learned to make camp and cook over a fire, to read a topographical map and route-find.

I was the oldest in the field by a decade and as such was viewed as a steadying presence. Consequently, I was assigned to share a tent with the youngest student, a sixteen-year-old girl named Katie. Katie hated everything about what we were doing. And she complained often about the long days of hiking. "It's just walking, Katie," I finally said to her one day in frustration. She just stared at me. The next evening, I was lying in our tent reading when I heard Katie and another student walking up. "We're just walking," Katie counseled the other student.

Then tragedy struck. While crossing a river, Katie slipped and fell. She hit her head on a rock, was swept downstream by the current, and was killed.

Several of us pulled her body from the water. The group's lead instructor, Liz, and I stayed close with Katie overnight, maintaining the fire in order to keep prey away. I remember feeling that the most important thing in the world that could have happened just happened, and yet the river rolled on, the forest still smelled of fragrant pine. The stars blazed in the night sky. In a strange way I felt privileged to be there. The following evening under a bloodred sunset a helicopter came in to retrieve Katie's body. The rest of us hiked out of the mountains over three long days.

In the weeks that followed, I loitered in Lander, not wanting or ready to just jump back into my life. Liz, the course instructor, and I grew close. We became lovers. Our relationship lasted six months. We have remained dear friends ever since—yet more than a year or two can easily go by without contact. I haven't seen her or returned to Lander in a dozen years.

A typical Wyoming working town of seven thousand, Lander life centers along Main Street. Other than a few more coffee shops, little has changed. Pickup trucks and Subarus glide by, capturing the schizophrenic nature of the place—ranchers and outdoor enthusiasts coexisting amiably.

I turn off Main Street onto Second. Then, on the corner of Eugene Street, I arrive at the small corner house with a picket fence. Liz and I initially grew close under profound and serious circumstances; our conversations have always bypassed the casual and gone directly to the core of the matter. And they do now. At the kitchen table we talk relationships, work, our kids—and it's this last that brings the most immediate news. Liz's daughter, Violet, is seventeen and transitioning.

"Violet's pronouns are *he* and *him*," Liz tells me by way of introduction to the topic. My recollection of Violet is of a small child with flowing hair and a Band-Aid on his knee, chasing Scout, the dog, around the backyard.

As Liz goes off to the market, I make a cup of weak tea, and Violet joins me at the kitchen table. He still has flowing brown hair and his mother's blue eyes. "There was this weird period when I was about ten," he begins. "I don't know what it was. I was like, 'I'm not comfortable being a girl, or addressed as such.' And the feelings grew."

A senior in high school now, Violet began taking testosterone eight months ago. "I've got more hair now, which is kind of dope, and my voice has gone a little lower. It'll really start to manifest sometime in this school year. I'll appear more masculine, so we're gonna see what happens with that."

"What bathroom do you use at school?"

"The girls'," Violet says matter-of-factly. "I'm just trying to pee, not prove anything."

"Must be a precarious moment for you," I say.

"Definitely," Violet says. "I mean, it's interesting growing up here. It's a very conservative place. When people find out, I'm pretty sure they won't talk to me anymore. 'Cause I know we can't connect well enough, because there's this part of me that they don't know, this part of me they'll dislike. So, it's tricky to make connections right now."

"Make you feel alone?"

"Hundred percent. It's pretty hard to make friends without being out to everybody. But I've talked to my parents a bunch about it, and close friends." He shrugs. "I can't fully share it with the rest of the place I'm in."

Violet is planning to take the name Boden. "I still present as female, but I consider myself male. I identify more with my male friends—that's a change in the past few years. It might be me trying to push away from more feminine things, but it definitely feels more comfortable for me to form deeper connections with guys. I have an easier time understanding my male friends."

And while we've been talking, Finn, one of those friends with whom Violet has a deeper connection, has walked in the back door. Finn was born male and identifies as such. With long hair and painted fingernails, he presents as fairly androgynous. The two have known each other their entire lives. "Our mothers were in the same prenatal class," Finn says, settling in with us at the kitchen table.

"Finn has an interesting position on masculinity and on friendship," Violet cues up his friend.

"I was instilled from an early age with this very Wyoming sense of masculinity," Finn explains. "The majority of my life I was plumb afraid of crying or to express emotion—that's not a man. I used to be really proud of how long it had been since I cried. I told Violet, 'It's been six years since I cried.' Violet looked at me and said, 'That's not good.' That one comment caused this spiral of introspection on why I felt this way and who was commanding me to feel this way.

"I realized this textbook Wyoming masculinity is going to leave me in the dust of loneliness. So I started questioning it. I'd sit in the dark and think, 'Am I happy with who I am? Do I feel that I'm a man?' And it's a conversation I've had several times as I've grown and gone through puberty. I think it's a conversation that's very valuable to have with yourself."

Violet looks across at his friend, nodding. "Finn and I talk about a lot of deep, intense stuff. I knew he was going to be chill with it when I told him what was going on."

Finn laughs. "I wasn't exactly like, 'Whoa, predicted it,' but it just connected some dots in my brain. 'This makes sense.' I could feel, especially in middle school, there was some tension that was unresolved."

"I was angsty," Violet concedes.

"You definitely had some aggression and internalized frustration I didn't understand."

Finn turns to me. "Look, being trans or questioning your identity is such a taboo topic, especially in Wyoming, and in this community... I mean, teachers have to tell your parents if you want to be called a different name than is on your birth certificate. They're required to blow the whistle on a student."

I sip my tea. "Grateful you two found each other?"

"Definitely," they say simultaneously.

"It's a lifeline," Violet goes on, "to know that I have these few people who I know will support me and I know no matter what happens, will be my friends continuously, that's pretty cool to have, and I think a lot of people don't have that. I feel super lucky to have made these connections."

"Violet and I are the closest of any friends in the school," Finn says with pride.

"Hell yeah!" Violet nearly shouts.

"I don't feel like I have to compromise any of my truest beliefs and truest morals and what makes me comfortable and what makes me flourish as a human being," Finn says. "I don't feel fear that any of me is going to be rejected."

"One hundred percent." Violet nods vigorously.

"I think I could get in Violet's car and just say whatever is on my mind and it would spark a conversation that is completely free of judgment and completely free of any awkwardness."

"We overshare so much!" Violet laughs. "Sometimes we try that with other people and they... don't do that."

The two friends find this hysterical.

"We're so lucky," Finn says, "that this grand cosmic roulette board matched his marble to my number or vice versa. That's how it feels. And it feels rare. And whether consciously or subconsciously, we recognize that. It's this incredible stroke of luck that I have him and he has me."

"We're good friends," Violet adds simply.

"If Violet somehow, God forbid, disappeared tomorrow"—Finn leans back—"I would still, on my deathbed, be like, that was such an important part of me and my life."

Violet looks at his friend. "Dope."

Wilson, Wyoming

The morning is bright and clear, the air mild—the kind of day when it feels things will always be this way. I have breakfast with Liz in one of the new coffee shops in town. We talk easily and deeply. Trading concerns and insights—a valuable use of time. Then she's off to work and I'm on the road.

I stop at the Sinclair gas station to fill my tank. When I restart the car, the radio is blaring—it wasn't on when I stopped the engine. A man is preaching about the light of God, the tree of light, the golden lamp of Moses, and stretching metaphors to the breaking point. I listen for a while, then flip the switch and return to blessed silence.

A few miles beyond Lander, heading west on the Chief Washakie Trail, a road I've driven numerous times over the decades, I pass a small sign I've never noticed. Doubling back, I head up an uneven track. A few miles and a few turns on unmarked roads and I arrive at a fairly large, very primitive cemetery filled mostly with wooden crosses on the slope of an exposed hillside, the foothills of the Wind River Mountains beyond. It's here that Sacagawea, the Native American guide and interpreter who accompanied Lewis and Clark across America, is buried. I had stumbled upon Meriwether Lewis's grave site way back in Tennessee while driving the bucolic Natchez Trace Parkway. Drawing a string between the two sites ties my trip together in a way that makes a kind of sense I can't explain to myself.

I wander slowly among the graves. The sun is bright, but a cool wind blows. My attention is taken by two horses, one chestnut, the other gray, standing side by side, head to tail, unmoving. A small white horse is lying motionless on the ground beside them, steps from the wooden crosses. I'm unable to locate Sacagawea's exact grave site and content myself with watching the two horses stand vigil over the third.

And I think of my friend Keith.

Keith was my first close friend to die. He was more than a friend. He was the only mentor I have ever had. In many ways, he saved my life—at least creatively.

In the wake of my early success in acting, and without consciously knowing I was looking, I went searching for answers. I began to travel the world. Alone. I didn't know at the time, but I was attempting to root myself by uprooting myself, trying to prove to myself that I was safe, both in the world and in who I was in myself.

One day, out of the blue, at a hotel in Saigon, I picked up a pen to write about an experience I had that day. Then for the next decade, whenever I was on the road, I did the same. I filled notebooks that gathered space on my shelves at home. One day I decided I wanted to do something with all those jottings, or at least with the experiences I had been gathering.

Through a work acquaintance, I met Keith. He was the editor-in-chief at *National Geographic Traveler* magazine, and after a year of my cajoling and pestering, he relented and let me write an article for him about Ireland, a place I knew well. This began a decade-long association. Keith taught me the game, the dos and don'ts, ins and outs. He sloughed off criticism from his colleagues who couldn't understand why he was investing in "some actor." Keith saw something in me I barely dared admit. In what may be odd advice from the editor of a travel magazine, he counseled me early on, "Don't be a travel writer. Be a writer who travels." He cheered my successes and prodded me to do better. We became friends.

A lion of a man, Keith was broad-shouldered with tufts of gray hair protruding above the open collar of his shirt, and I knew more than a few writers who were terrified of him. Several years into our association, we were having breakfast at one of those grand New York hotels he loved to pretend to hate, when he confessed in very simple terms how much fear he experienced in his daily life and how he felt he couldn't allow it to show. Keith was well aware of my own journey through fear via travel—I had written about it often enough for him. I understood instantly Keith's experience of fear as a chronic condition, not an acute reaction to circumstances. Fear, I knew, was content to feed upon itself. We talked about the feelings of shame that often accompany such fear, especially for a man. We spoke of our shared history of abusing alcohol—how the drink had pushed that fear and shame away, at least for a time, until the alcohol invariably turned those feelings inward and compounded them.

At his memorial service, others eulogized Keith's formidable reputation and his love for his children. I highlighted this breakfast and how close it made me feel to my mentor, how human it made him, how fortunate I felt to be trusted. After, people approached me with surprise, even disbelief, to hear that Keith had admitted to such feelings of frailty.

I back away and leave the wooden crosses and horses and wind and turn my sights to my friend John, a few hours to the west.

John and I first met in a conference room of the Pronghorn Lodge in Lander, for something called a critical incident stress debrief. It was several days after the tragedy in which Katie had died crossing the river. John was the head of the Rocky Mountain branch of the outdoor school that ran the trip. Everyone who had been in any way connected with the course sat in a large circle to talk through their experience of the event. John led the session. Robust and blond, he looked every inch the mountaineering outdoorsman. He handled the session head-on and with compassion.

As I hung around Lander those next few months with Liz, I would occasionally run into John. Something in his manner attracted me. He was the kind of person I'd like to be friends with, I told myself. We stayed vaguely in touch, and several years later he reached out when coming to New York. We got together for a drink and decided we'd take a trip into the outdoors together. It took several more years to pull it off, but we finally met to go canoeing down the Green River in Utah. I was excited by the prospect, but it triggered my latent fear—that I wasn't man enough in the world. And now I was headed out into the wilderness with a man who had summited Himalayan peaks.

We had several enjoyable days of paddling and sleeping under the stars, then John began to grow remote. My insecurities got the best of me, and I was sure he was wondering what the hell he was doing out in the wilderness with this "wimp." Finally, I confronted the issue. John had no idea what I was talking about. In fact, the situation was the exact opposite.

John was carrying a long-held secret, and since he was growing to trust me and appreciate my perspectives, he was preparing to unburden himself. I listened to his secret, then shrugged and said, "Well, dude, this has happened to better men than you." He bristled, but it burst a bubble of isolation and exclusivity he had been living in, and a friendship was born.

We continued to go out into the wilderness every few years, backpacking into Wind River Mountains, we scaled the South Teton together, and we took our kids canoeing through the Missouri Breaks in Montana. Somewhere along the way, my fear that I just wasn't man enough faded to the point that I failed to consider it much anymore. This friendship was largely responsible for that.

On one visit to New York, John stayed with my family. One night, we were eating alone and he said to me, "I can really feel the strain." John was referring to how I carried the responsibilities of family life. I was embarrassed by the accuracy of his remark—much as he had bristled at mine to him years earlier. But it was liberating.

I realized in that moment how self-indulgent my behavior had been, how I had used the perceived strain to push away those closest to me. To isolate myself. It also came clear to me that I'd been looking for some imagined person or committee, some phantom "grown-up," to honor me for my unique sacrifice. John's comment made me see the folly, the childishness of that as well. I was simply living the life I'd created. Yes, I had very real responsibilities, but they were typical—and so was I. John's calling out my self-glorified struggle altered how I accepted and viewed those responsibilities, and consequently how I related to those closest to me, and how I moved through the world.

Crossing the Continental Divide now, the sun hits hard off the Pinnacle Buttes of the Absaroka Mountains and then I'm up and over Togwotee Pass at 9,655 feet, the Teton Range coming into view for the first time. "Wow," I say aloud, and laugh—the way I always do whenever I first glimpse the Tetons, jutting abruptly from the golden valley floor to nearly 14,000 jagged, postcard-ready feet.

It takes another hour to reach the town of Jackson, which, in the quarter century I've been coming here, has in many ways become a victim of its own success. Range Rovers have largely supplanted pickup trucks. At the Cowboy Coffee Company, puffer coats have displaced Wrangler jackets. High-priced Western-themed art fills the shops lining the town square. Traffic jams are not uncommon, even between seasons like I am now.

Past town, I make a few turns off North Moose-Wilson Road, and then I'm on gravel, driving through bare aspens and rounding a bend to John's two-story, chinked log cabin.

Because John's and my friendship is one born in adulthood and not youth, I've occasionally felt its roots did not go as deep. There have been spans of time when we didn't speak for a few years at a stretch, and I thought that perhaps our friendship had run its course.

"There are some friendships that exist for a certain period and serve a certain function," I say to John after we've settled around the idle firepit surrounded by aspen and pine. A small creek runs close by. "I've thought at times that our friendship was one of those. Not that those friendships have to end badly or over a falling-out, but life just moves on."

"I've wondered that as well," John says. "I'm glad it hasn't."

We hear a sound and turn. A large bull elk slowly picks a path through the brush on the other side of the stream, twenty feet away. We watch in silence, then sit still in the wake of that.

Still looking off, John says, "I remember when I was getting divorced, you and I were talking several times a week, and you called me one day to check in while I was shoveling snow, clearing the driveway. I was having a really hard time, and you said, 'Just keep shoveling, dude.'"

I laugh. "Genius, huh?"

"No, really. To this day, whenever I'm struggling with something, that's my mantra."

"Well, I'm not the first to say something like that."

John looks across at me. "But you were there to say it, dude." Then, because he has an analytical mind that likes to categorize things, John contextualizes our friendship in what he calls his "rings of friendship."

"There's the inner circle. The guys I'd trust with my deepest failures, my concerns, my inadequacies. They have my deepest trust. They tend to be ones I've gone through hardship with in some way, but I don't hang with them much. I'd say there are four in that circle. You're in that circle."

I inwardly smile like a schoolkid chosen on the playground—then silently ask myself when exactly will I grow up?

"Then there's another circle," John goes on, unaware of my inner childishness. "I'll do hardship with them, but I'll be a little more guarded on some aspect of my life. That ring has many more players in it. They're more than acquaintances—I'd call them up and do something with them. Then there are those folks I see at parties, I give them a big hug, I'd connect with them, then we'll go away. I don't make plans with them."

I can see the Grand Teton through the bare trees. Wisps of clouds trail off its northern face. The sky around it is a brilliant blue. Winter is coming to the mountains.

John looks around. "Just today, I was sitting out here, 'cause I can't do anything right now with this shoulder, and I was watching, the trees, birds, the animals. I thought, 'This is the nicest part of my day.' And I realized that I've become more energized by watching rather than doing. I'm less motivated by achievement. And ambition, for sure."

"That coming from an achievement-oriented guy," I say.

He nods. "Identity for me has been a big thing. How am I known? I'm this outdoor guy. But I've realized I'm not looking for a legacy. Those things in the end are easily forgotten. I'm not interested in that now. I am interested in experiences with people who are important to me."

John shifts to accommodate his just-operated-on shoulder.

"How's that shoulder feeling?" I ask.

"You know what's harder than the physical discomfort. Not being able to do stuff for myself right now."

"You mean you have trouble asking for help? Get in line with that one, dude."

He laughs. "I'm really uncomfortable letting Jinny do all these things for me now, 'cause of this shoulder. Admitting a weakness," he says.

"The fact that your wife loves you and is happy to help you doesn't matter?"

"You tell him, Andrew," Jinny says, appearing from behind us and taking a seat.

Later, John and I are out walking his dog. We talk about our kids. We talk about how money is never really just about money. We talk about the slippery slope of alcohol. We talk about the relief it feels to talk so freely.

Again and again on this trip, I'm amazed that I can turn up in a seemingly random place and sit down with someone I haven't seen and have hardly spoken to, sometimes in years, and launch right in on personal and intimate details of our lives.

Over dinner the following evening, accompanied by Jinny, I mention how the word "trust" has come up repeatedly in the conversations I've been having with men.

"Trust is interesting," John says. "People often say trust is built over time. And I think that's true. But it doesn't have to work that way. I trusted you with something I'd never told anyone, something I'd been carrying, and we didn't know each other well at all at that point. And I don't know why I did. It was just this feeling that I could trust you."

"Spidey sense."

"Yeah, exactly. And trust is an easier word than some others," John goes on. "Trust implies, 'I got your back, you got mine.' Manly stuff. But you gotta walk through the door of vulnerability to get to trust."

"And there's the rub," I say.

"Vulnerability has a landscape in a lot of different forms. From just being somewhat open, to the far end of shedding tears, and that scares men. Men aren't vulnerable because they're afraid of being shamed."

I mention Derek and Joe in Sedona, how they referred to that same sense of shame. Then jokingly I ask, "What do you think a Wyoming cowboy would say about that?"

"That's easy," Jinny says. "I can connect you with one."

Jackson Hole, Wyoming

Which leads me to Cody.

A fifth-generation Jackson native, Cody's family's ranch is the largest provider of beef in the valley, with a stunning expanse of land on the edge of town.

"How many head of cattle do you run?" I ask, getting off on the wrong foot.

"Enough to eat the grass," Cody says curtly.

Taking the bait and stepping further into manure, I inquire, "How many acres of grass you got?"

"Enough to feed the cows."

Then Cody softens. Slightly.

"That's like askin' a banker how much money he has in his account. We just don't do that around here."

"Should I leave now?"

Cody concedes the slightest smile from under his mustache. Forty, with graying temples and pale blue eyes that match his Wrangler jeans and Wrangler shirt snapped to the collar, wearing brown boots and in possession of a brown cowboy hat, Cody looks every inch the American cowboy.

"I grew up with cowboys and you wanted to make sure everyone knew you were tough as hell. That's how you ate your lunch, how you got in and out of your truck, how you took care of your horse. It's just a stoic thing. That's how you present yourself."

Cody takes a seat behind the modern glass desk in his minimalist office—minimalist save for the head of a Rocky Mountain Longhorn ram and one of a Herford bull mounted on the walls.

He's quick to recite for me the unwritten code of the West. "'Live each day with courage. Take pride in your work. Always finish what you start. Do what has to be done. Be tough but fair. If you make a promise, keep it. Ride for the brand. Talk less, say more. Remember some things are not for sale. Know where to draw the line.'"

"That sounds good," I say, then chance getting kicked out again, "as far as it goes."

Cody eyes me narrowly. "All that basically says is, be stoic. I grew up with that philosophy, and at some point I made an effort to be a quiet man."

"You have kids?" I ask, looking for a way in.

"Two. Six and four years old." He smiles.

Cody has also volunteered with the Jackson Hole Search and Rescue team for the past fourteen years, leading it for the past seven. "I've extracted people from an avalanche dead and had to tell their families. I come from a generation where you just pull your hat down when that happens and move on with your day, don't show weakness. And that's maybe a healthy way to handle it. But on the other hand, in Search and Rescue we're educated on a lot of mental health stuff. You learn that just pulling your hat down is creating garbage that your wife is gonna have to deal with, that your kids are gonna have to deal with.

"You gotta work through it, talk through it. Some of that knowledge helps me lift the veil a bit and realize it's okay to be vulnerable. In fact, it creates closer relationships with people when you show that vulnerability. At end of day, it makes life easier."

I watch Cody wrestle with this notion in silence. Then he says, "We've all seen those mountain hardmen who after twenty years have those hollow eyes. People who became too jaded to function well in society."

"Or put a bullet in their head," I say.

"I've seen that too." Cody nods. "For that very reason. I know what that looks like and know I can have some tendencies toward that myself, so…"

I'm conscious not to display any reaction to that remark.

Then Cody's internal pendulum swings back. "Still, you want to have that grit. Being open and vulnerable, it's something I'm working on. But I couldn't go to the rancher next door, or a cowboy working for us, and tell him I'm feelin' this or that, 'cause that would come across as weakness. They'd think, 'This guy can't handle it.'

"My brother Casey, for example, he's a super hard-ass. He's on Search and Rescue also. And if he just dug a kid out of the mountain, I know what he's going through. But then if there's one person you gotta be tough with, it's your brother."

I wonder if this is another part of some personal code—does toughness equate to love? Do those you love the most need to be treated the toughest?

"It's tricky," Cody goes on. "It's not like we've figured out how to be an open vulnerable person and a hard-ass at the same time. 'Cause I haven't."

"You have a friend who you're closest with?"

"Twenty years ago, I would have said I had a best friend, but not now." He considers his hands, folded on the desktop. "My best friend growing up still lives in town. I see him a time or two a year. You'd think 'cause we live in the same town we'd see each other, but we've each got our lives, got our professions. We don't drop in every Sunday to watch football.

"I did go elk hunting a while back with my friend Ryan. Sleeping three feet apart, spending six days, essentially holding hands. I mean we talked about life a little, but mostly it was 'Where do you think the bear is?' or 'Are you tired?' My relationships are based on activities like that."

Like so many men I've spoken with on this topic, after an initial reluctance, Cody's interested to explore the subject. "I've always taken my friendships for granted. But as I've gotten older, I'm starting to understand the things that help me function well as a man, as a human—and having good relations is part of it."

"So, you're cultivating those relationships?"

He shrugs. "Well, my wife handles our social calendar."

"Do you have friendships with women?"

"No."

We sit.

"I appreciate the idea of the American cowboy. It stands for a lot of things that resonate with me. It's more than just the hat. It's what I want my identity to be—whether that's real or not I don't know yet."

"Fair enough," I say.

"But I do know the toughest bull gets the girl, it's that simple. I watch it happen. The biggest ram lives the highest on the mountain by himself. That's real, I'm not making it up. But I also see how that doesn't lead to a super happy existence. So, is the goal of a man to be happy or tough? I go back and forth on that one."

"You want your kids to be happy or tough?"

"I want them to be tough," Cody says without having to consider the point. "Toughness is a defining thing, central to our value."

"Cowboy up."

"Cowboy up." Cody nods. "I say it to my kids all the time. It's something I was preached, and generally I like that ideal—toughen up, bear down, get it done. A 'do what has to be done' mentality. But I will say, as that attitude meets the modern world, it's not always smooth interaction. I can't say 'Cowboy up' in public anymore. Not everyone sees that as a universally appropriate way to handle the world. And as I've said, I can see how that philosophy has led to some discontent, some unhappiness in life. We're at a crossroads of society. When's the right time to cowboy up and when's the right time to pour it out? Finding the right balance, that's the challenge, that's the yin and yang of it.

"And look, to be sincere, to be a straight shooter, you can't just act tough, act like you have it together, or act like nothing's wrong if something obviously is. 'Cause that's not sincere, that's not being a bull, that's not genuine. So maybe what being a cowboy is..." Cody falters and looks around the room, then out the window at the world he inherited and takes pride in, a world he's keen to perpetuate. "...It evolves." Cody trains his blue eyes on me. "What is being a man? It's changed."

Don

Boise, Idaho

Once over the 8,432-foot Teton Pass I'm into Idaho, heading west and finally toward Don. Past tiny Victor, then through pleasant Idaho Falls, the land flattens and dries and dries and flattens some more. If you were looking for a place to put a nuclear facility in the 1950s, what came to be known as Atomic City, on little-used Route 26, would have been a good spot. But when reactor SL-1 exploded and killed three men on January 3, 1961, it became the site of the first nuclear accident in America. Not much remains today but wind and sky, a few derelict buildings, and a gas station doubling as a bar. A little farther on is Arco, whose claim to fame is that it was the first "city" in the world to be lit by atomic power. In truth, there's not much to light.

I chitchat with Seve on the phone while eating an appropriately overcooked Atomic Burger (fries extra) at Pickle's Place on Front Street. Then I'm back on the road. Past the lava rock fields of the Craters of the Moon National Monument, I'm in the mood to just keep going. But when I'm shoved onto I-84 with the interstate's quota of heedless trucks, I've had enough and limp my way into Boise wondering why I drove so far west when my intent was to dip down into Nevada sooner. But as I've discovered on this trip, there are times, especially the longer I'm out here, that the road tells me where to go.

Boise is having a moment. Its population is young, it's close to the outdoors, its downtown is buzzing and walkable. The avenues are wide and parking is easy. I wander the de rigueur promenade containing the standard array of bars and restaurants.

On the corner of West Idaho and Eleventh Street, I slip into the Record Exchange, an oasis of vinyl—pop, rock, rap, country, classical, jazz, blues, all laid out in old-fashioned record bins. It's got a tiny café. It sells toothbrushes. The place is a sanctuary for music geeks, misfits, and a weary traveler who hasn't owned a turntable since the 1990s. My shoulders relax, and I wander idly, feeling suddenly received in Boise.

It's between the spoken word and the blues that I encounter a middle-aged man with a trim goatee and an open face tucked under a baseball cap. Jimmy has managed this place since 1990, not long after arriving in Boise from Oregon. He met his wife here, raised a kid here—he's an easy guy to chat with, and he knows it.

"I'm not that judgmental. I'm accepting of things that might be annoying. I can get along with anybody, but men's men, locker-room talk, that shit has turned me off as long as I can remember. And I like women. I'm friends with as many women as men. And I stay friends for a long time."

Jimmy and I make our way over to one of the half dozen fifties-style vinyl booths snug under the windows with a view out onto Eleventh Street.

"Women listen differently," he goes on. "They talk differently. They're collaborative, inclusive. Men tend to want to be 'the man,' driving forward, digging down into one thing. Women can luxuriate in details, and it drives men crazy. But I like tangents.

Conversation with women can be a lot of tangents. And it's inclusive. I'm generalizing, of course. I know many women who are hyper-focused as well. But generally speaking…"

A young coworker in a Dolly Parton T-shirt comes by the booth, asking if that 1950s black hot rod parked outside is mine. I assure him it's not. He then asks Jimmy for help with something at the register.

"You can figure that out, Tim. If you can't, come back." The young man walks off. Jimmy smiles to himself and gazes out the window before continuing.

"That John Wayne archetype," Jimmy says, "it runs on fear. Everything runs on fear, fear of being homeless, fear of the other. It's hardwired into us. We are such a social species, but we're looking for people like us.

"The whole 'lone wolf' is a myth that should die. You look around at some point and it's like 'where is everybody?' Then you get mad about the fact that nobody conforms to the roles you've set up for them in your head as a lone wolf. You get pissed off at that motherfucker—'I'm gonna kill him. They're not conforming to what I've decided in my head alone.'

"You spend too much time in your own mind, it starts playing weird tricks—that's not good. I like being in my head, and trying to sort things out, but only to a certain point can you do that before you need input.

"'What do you do?' is often the opening gambit in the manosphere. But that's fair enough. With men, we've experienced the same things, the same pressures. And what's implicit in that question? Pro-vi-ding—" He divides the word into three heavy sections, endowing it with the weight of thirty years' obligation on it.

Talking with Jimmy in such quick succession after Cody in Jackson, I'm struck not only by how many ways there are for a man to inhabit the world, but how the weight of the obligation to provide feels so universal and ingrained. And as John pointed out to me years ago, our relationship to that weight goes a long way in dictating how we as men navigate the world.

Jimmy's coworker in the Dolly Parton T-shirt returns. "Got it figured out," he says and keeps moving.

"Great," Jimmy says to Tim's retreating figure. Jimmy turns back to me. "It's good for humans to not feel like you're alone. You're out there, winging it, but knowing that you can show up on your friend's doorstep and they'd get a blanket out for you—that's cool. I've been exceedingly fortunate. The people that I've collected are true. They're stalwarts. They don't tell you what to do, you don't tell them, but you can share your experience, and if you have anything to offer, you offer it. That broadens your experience, broadens your palate. It hooks you in with the thing that is bigger than yourself. And that's important. We run into problems when we deny that need."

Jimmy takes his cap off and runs his hand through what gray hair remains. "I'm 'the record store guy,' and that's all right. That's enough. People know me around town, and I like that. I'm connected. And that connection is huge. I stand behind that counter every day. Come on by."

I find a certain nobility in Jimmy's position.

"I just have to make the rest of it count for something," he concludes. "Embrace the people I know and love, charge my phone, come to work every day, grind it out, see what happens."

Later, a few blocks away at the Modern Motel, I approach the skinny man with a buzz cut and granny glasses behind the counter and ask for a room. He groans, "Nnnn, I don't know," and swivels to his computer. "I don't think we have anything left." He hits a few more keys without much hope.

"Jimmy from the record store sent me, said this was the place to stay."

The man looks up over his glasses. "Jimmy sent you?"

"He did."

"I think I might have one room left."

The next morning I'm over at Goldy's Breakfast Bistro, a nook of a place, at a table beside a father and his teenage son. When they finish ordering, the waiter, a tall and bearded hipster with a good attitude and a sleeve of tattoos, compliments them on their choices. "Nice order, guys!" he enthuses and scoops up the menus. "Well done." The father and son, left alone, say nothing. Each stares at his water glass. Maybe I just haven't had my tea yet, or maybe all my conversations have begun to illuminate something for me in the need each man feels and how ill-equipped we so often seem to meet or even identify that need.

An hour south of Boise on Highway 51, brown hills slowly begin to push their way up, first into random bumps and then the land begins to roll. Then I'm in grassland. There are no other cars. Glancing at the speedometer, I'm going a hundred miles an hour. Up in the hills as I come out of a bend, I'm forced to brake hard for a man crossing a dozen head of cattle. He offers a lazy wave. Recently scorched trees line the left of the narrow road. Unmarred grassland extends off on the right.

Then I'm across the forty-second parallel, cutting through the Duck Valley Indian Reservation. The road hugs the tight curves of the Owyhee River through the valley. I'm in Nevada. A sign tells me it's one hundred miles to the next gas in Elko. Beyond that tired town, I continue south, on Route 278. Seve calls to break up the monotony.

"Where are you now?"

"I'm the only one on some random road in northern Nevada."

"Lonely out there?"

"Actually, I'm loving it." Then I challenge my friend. "How about you? Lonely?"

I'm prepared for a deflection, for Seve to talk about whatever game is on television tonight and how he's looking forward to that. But he surprises me.

"Well, I'm grateful for you and Eddie."

I consider this and decide to push a bit. "If we were in a court of law, I'd say you didn't answer the question."

We laugh.

"Well, I'm housebound right now, so I'd normally give you a different answer."

"I'll buy that," I say.

"But I do feel, talking to you and Eddie, I feel connected. And I don't feel connected to a lot of people."

Seve is rarely so open and direct in addressing his feelings. But the safety of the phone, the distance, plus our familiarity with the topic over numerous conversations on this trip all allow an ease to our back and forth. Seve's intermittent riding long-distance shotgun beside me on this journey has been a happy surprise and form of support for us both. And right now he's feeling relaxed and safe. "I can pick up the phone and feel connected quickly because of our legacy. I think back to New York, and I have no idea how we became bonded to each other."

"No idea." I laugh. "But we are."

"I've always felt you said what was on your mind. And I never felt judged," he says. "From the beginning. We speak truth to each other. I'm safe in that. We trust each other."

"Agreed."

"And the great thing is that when I talk to you, to Eddie, I feel like I'm still growing."

That last comment, made in Seve's offhanded way, is a powerful thing to say about friendship. One I'd never considered. I look out over the narrow road, long and flat and straight, rushing under the car. The sky is a miracle of blue. The simplicity and possibility contained in Seve's remark, the open-ended quality of it, is enough to fill that space.

We ride together in silence for a time. Then Seve asks after my kids. I mention something I said to my daughter on the phone earlier, about her commitment to schoolwork, that's been gnawing at me.

Seve sighs. "I know that tone of voice."

"What?" I demand, suddenly defensive.

"I know what you mean when you say what you said to Willow. And I don't think you're wrong. But you saying that face-to-face, when she can see you and feel your love and empathy, and you saying that on the phone in that tone you just used with me—you are saying two very different things."

I'm silent. The desert whips by, sage and dirt and rock. "Well, shit." He's right.

Seve mentions something about his beloved Baltimore Orioles.

"Stop bothering me," I snap. "I gotta go call my daughter."

"Love ya, pal."

"Yeah, yeah, love ya bye," and I hang up fast.

Eureka, Nevada

In 1864, three silver miners wandered into Horse Thief Canyon looking for a quiet place to dig. They struck silver, and the boom was on. A hundred twenty-five saloons, as well as twenty-five gambling halls, sprang up to service men working fifty mines and a population of ten thousand. Then within twenty-five years it was mostly over.

Today, with less than four hundred souls remaining, there's not exactly a buzz around Eureka, Nevada, but the three active mines still spit out enough gold nuggets to sustain a faint pulse. Eureka offers up an easy, if unpolished, welcome in the middle of a desperate desert. Several Victorian buildings from the 1870s, including the Opera House and Jackson Hotel, remain.

A handwritten sign on the glass door of the hotel advises me to head to the more recently built motel on the edge of town to arrange a stay here. So I do.

"You want to stay at the Jackson?" the young lady behind the counter of the motel asks. She seems surprised.

"Is there availability?" I ask.

"Oh yes." She nods. "There's just one guest staying there, one of the miners."

"Great," I say. "One night, please."

She hesitates. "Okay." She shuffles some papers. "You don't want to stay here?"

"This is nice," I say, looking around the largely fiberboard lobby with plastic finishes. "That just looks like a cool old place."

"Oh, it is. I love it there."

"Perfect."

She sets about the paperwork. Her name is Netta. She's in her late twenties. After a minute, Netta looks up. "It's haunted. You know that, right?"

"Oh?"

"I just thought you should know."

"Seriously?"

"Oh, yes."

"Ghosts?"

"Mmm-hmm." She nods.

"Have you seen them?"

"I feel them." She smiles to herself and leans toward me, confiding, "I sense things other people don't." Netta has small teeth. Her mousy hair is pulled back tight against her scalp. "But tons of people have had encounters."

"I see. How often do you 'sense' them?"

"Every time I go up to change the sheets and stuff."

"So not just at night."

"Oh, no, anytime. They're quite active."

"Okay. Well...what ghosts are there?"

"There's an eleven-year-old girl—she likes to do pranks on people. And the lady in red—she used to work in the brothel. She gets into bed with the guests."

"Does she do anything with them?" My mind begins to race.

"No, no. She just lays beside them in the bed."

"Too bad."

"And there's a cowboy, you hear him walking around, up and down the stairs a lot."

I'm not exactly sure what to do with this information. It's not that I do or don't believe in ghosts, but if ever there was a town where the paranormal might be hanging around, Eureka feels like the place. "Are they friendly?" I ask.

"Oh, yes. I just thought you should know."

Forewarned and forearmed, I head back up the road, unlock the door, climb a flight of stairs, and find my room. The Victorian room is a beautiful re-creation of ye olde times—wrought iron bed, glass lamp, lace curtains. It has a claw-foot bath.

I lie down on the bed to get a twenty-minute siesta after the long drive. I close my eyes. In short order I hear a creak. My eyes pop open.

"Hello?" I call out.

There's no response. I close my eyes again. I'm almost asleep when I think I hear a noise in the hall. I bolt upright. Now I'm freaking myself out. I go to the bathroom, telling myself I'm being childish. It's an old house. Old houses make a lot of noises. My phone rings and I jump, peeing all over the seat.

It's Seve again. He has another thought on the topic of friendship we were discussing earlier. I don't give him a chance—telling him where I am and what's happening.

"Are you crazy?" he says. "Didn't you see *The Shining*?"

"That really doesn't help," I tell him, but it's all I need to hear. I'm down the stairs and back at the motel up the road in five minutes. Netta doesn't blink when I return. She hands me a keycard to a generic room, and while I'm swiping the door my wife calls.

I fill her in on the past half hour, including Seve's remark.

"Andrew," Dolores says flatly, "there are no such things as ghosts."

"I saw *The Shining*!" I shout into the receiver.

I can hear her eye roll across the distance. "You and Seve deserve each other."

After a shower and a cup of tea, I've returned to myself enough to get something to eat. There are only two places in town, and the Urban Cowboy bar is closed this Sunday afternoon. Three doors up is the Owl Club—billing itself as a steakhouse. I settle for the burger.

"Get any good roadkill on your way into town?"

I look up from my French fries to the man turning around from the table in front of me. He's solidly built, stocky, topped with close-cropped gray hair on a square head. Large silver bangles seem an unlikely adornment on each wrist.

"Huh?" I say stupidly.

"You get any good roadkill on the way in? I got a couple of jackrabbits and a skunk."

"No, I didn't."

"They were tasty. Brought 'em in and they cooked 'em right up for me."

"What?"

"Yeah, delicious."

"Really?"

"You're in deep Nevada here. Most small towns, you take your roadkill, they'll prepare it for you. They made me a nice dinner."

"You stopped and picked up your roadkill?"

"Sure."

"And they prepared it?" I'm trying to take this in. "They made a stew?"

"Meat loaf."

"Didn't they have to skin them?"

"Well, they were already partly skinned." He smiles. "And gutted."

"Right." I nod, getting a visual I don't want. "What's skunk taste like?"

"Little gamey, but they mixed them together."

This is Howard. Aside from a table of two bikers across the room and a lone miner in the corner, we're the only ones in the place. The last of the sun's rays slash into the room. Dust motes float. Several unattended slot machines blink in the corner. Howard is a Nevada native, living now in northwest Washington. He's passing back through on his way to Mexico.

"It was time for me to get out of Dodge," he says. "Get away from people, find some solace. I need the sun. It's too wet and dark up in Washington, not good for my depression."

"You get depressed?"

"For years now."

"You take medication for that?"

"Oh, yeah."

"You see a shrink?"

"No. I did for a while when I got back from Iraq, but once I got it off my chest I stopped."

"What did you need to get off your chest?"

Howard served twenty-two years in the Army Corps of Engineers as a hydrographic surveyor—he talks at some length of his disillusionment with the military. "I thought we were in Iraq to help," he concludes. "I was wrong. I just took it personally. Made me bitter."

We're silent for a moment before Howard continues. "I had a friend there. If it weren't for him…" His thought goes unfinished.

"You stay in touch?"

"Oh yeah, we talk on the phone." Then he confesses, "But not much. It was a situational friendship."

I nod.

Howard goes on. "Never really had close friends. That didn't work for me. I did things that didn't involve friends. I hid a lot of feelings and issues behind macho stuff and ego. I was very isolated, didn't know who to talk to."

"You're talking about it pretty easily now with me."

"I'm old. I don't care anymore."

"You married, Howard?"

"Forty years."

"You talk to your wife about stuff?"

He shakes his head. "I never really talked to my wife."

"You find that isolating?"

"Oh, yeah."

"Must be for her too."

"The whole gender thing has gotten out of hand. Men don't know what to do anymore, don't know what women want. You don't know who you're going to offend. I'm pegged as an old white, racist male, and that's so far from the truth." Howard says all this in an amiable, accessible tone. "People like the dogma. But they have no idea who we are, who I am."

He gets up. I've enjoyed his offhanded candor and I'm sorry to see him go.

"You were joking about the roadkill, right?"

Howard smiles and pats my shoulder.

Across the street from the Owl is Louie's Lounge, *"Where the fun is"*—except there's not much fun to be had. Louie's looks to have closed down years ago. Likewise, the crumbling and abandoned hotel beside it—but at three stories, still the tallest building in town. What I do find open is the optimistically named Phoenix convenience store. And behind the counter stands a tall twenty-six-year-old, with patchy facial hair and a surprisingly fatalistic air of self-awareness. From down the road a few hours in Stagecoach, Mark's been in town just over two years. When I inquire about what a young fella does for fun in this nearly deserted mining town, he says brightly, "I go trail riding."

"Mountain bike?"

"In my Jeep, I got thirty-six-inch wheels. And I shoot at the range."

"What do you got?" I ask.

"I got a G-Force Arms pump-action shotgun."

And then I ask a version of the question I've asked so often on this trip. "Any friends around town?"

"I'd say more acquaintances," Mark replies simply. "I don't hang out with them outside of work. I stick to myself."

"Live with anyone?"

"My brother Dave."

It turns out Mark's brother Dave is not in fact his brother.

"Family is not just blood," Mark clarifies for me. Mark and Dave met four years ago. "We just clicked. We started as friends and became brothers—what most male friendships turn out to be if you're willing to give it your personal trust. If you don't, you're just acquaintances."

I consider the simplicity of this youthful certainty. And Mark goes on. "He's twenty-four. I call him my big little brother, 'cause he's six foot eight. It's an attitude we share. We're gonna make sure we get to where we want to get."

"Where do you want to get?"

Mark smiles and shifts his weight. Maybe he's not entirely sure yet, or maybe he is. "My own home. Three cars, a wife. The American dream, right? But without the picket fence. I don't want a picket fence."

When Mark's house burned down in an electrical fire, Dave, who works the mine, called his friend to come out and join him in Eureka.

"He said it was more peaceful. I didn't think I needed anyone. I was able to do things myself—I get knocked down and I get myself up and wipe my feet off." Mark shrugs. "But I get lonely a lot. Nothing happens. It's just how I feel sometimes. It's a random occurrence." He considers. "So, I came out here. It's better with a friend. We talk a lot, make sure the other's good. He comes by here and checks up on me."

Across America, from Maryland to Nevada, I've found the younger men I've met are easily, and without shame, willing to admit their loneliness, and not simply "pull the hat down."

"Better than being a lone wolf, huh?" I ask, expecting an easy yes in response. Instead, Mark offers a more complex reply.

"Depends where you are in life. People who I trusted broke my trust, and if I can't trust anybody, I'd rather I just got myself. You can't just let anyone in. They'll act like your friend but secretly put you down. A real friend celebrates your successes, but with fake friends they'll hope for your downfall." Mark says all this simply, an accepted fact. "There'll always be somebody degrading you—you don't need that in friendship. You gotta have respect and trust. They go hand in hand. You don't respect each other you're not gonna get anywhere. Sometimes me and Dave talk about how lucky we are to have each other, how grateful we are. Sometimes you need to hear that."

I tell Mark I agree with him.

He smiles. "He just kind of popped up. I was okay where I was, but sometimes friends just pop up."

We both stand briefly in satisfied silence.

"We're all we got right now," Mark concludes.

Lake Tahoe, California
Part 2

Heading west out of Eureka, the two lanes of US Route 50 cut straight across central Nevada, with only a few fragile settlements strung along its course, hours apart. A geographic pattern emerges as you drive through this part of the Great Basin. Long, flat periods of ruler-straight road unfold until you come upon once distant mountains. The road then rises and bends, navigating the most forgiving undulations through the mountains. It then descends back onto the high plane, where another set of distant mountains can be made out on the horizon. The road straightens itself out until it comes upon those mountains and then up it goes, bending and twisting, before descending and straightening. It goes on like this for hours. The land flanking the road is stark, majestic for its lack of allure, regal in its sense of absence. What vegetation there is consists mainly of sagebrush steppe. The road grows deeply comforting in its certainty. In 1986, *LIFE* magazine dubbed Highway 50 "the loneliest road in America." I've been looking forward to driving it since I knew I was headed to see Don.

The thing about Route 50 is that since being crowned with such a provocative title, it now draws a crowd—well, "crowd" is a bit rich. But with the camper vans and bikers who traverse it, there is a steady, if light, flow. I've driven far more lonely stretches of road over the past weeks. Long stretches of the twisting

Appalachian roads felt abandoned. The desolate, daunting Chihuahuan Desert in West Texas stands out. Parts of eastern Utah felt more remote. Southwestern Wyoming was very quiet and exposed. Even coming down from Idaho and into northern Nevada felt more isolated. Yet despite fame having robbed Route 50 of some of its solitude, it is still a profound and singular stretch of the American West.

I'd anticipated a feeling of relief upon reentering conventional and familiar society, yet I find myself disappointed to reach Fallon, knowing that from here to the California coast I will not encounter such untrammeled earth again.

Time after time I've experienced the oft-documented feeling of freedom and possibility the open road inspires, the whispered promise, the sense of exhilaration that comes from taking a rise and seeing mile upon mile of open range and undeveloped land. "The space," I've gasped aloud stupidly more than a few times, entranced, impotently trying to capture for myself the awe the West inspires.

And it's not just the West, but across America, my kneejerk dislike of driving has often been transformed by the physical beauty I've encountered in so many of its forms, inspiring head-shaking wonder. But such warm thoughts are quickly brushed aside as I'm forced onto the six lanes of I-80 at Sparks, Nevada. A Jeep spewing black exhaust passes me on the right, then swerves in front. The usual array of eighteen-wheelers roar. I hunch my shoulders.

A fast exit onto Route 431 and just as quickly I'm among the pine, climbing Mount Rose. I gain elevation and crest a pass at 8,900 feet. Snow is in evidence—soon this pass may not be open.

The view east takes in Reno and Sparks. To the west are the Sierra Nevada. The road plummets, and sooner than expected I'm on the north shore of shimmering Lake Tahoe.

I spent time here decades earlier with Seve and Eddie. Youthful, reckless fun. Hugging the lake and just over the border into California, I pull off to take a photo in front of the sign for Kings Beach. It was here that Seve met a girl—the kind of memory accompanied by a shudder.

On the morning we were to leave Tahoe, and after days of searching for Seve, who had gone AWOL, Eddie and I found him in Kings Beach, shacked up in a trailer park. "Go home without me. I'm staying," Seve called through the door as we pounded on the trailer at dawn. "Juss leave me," he slurred.

We didn't.

I text the photo of the sign, with no caption, to both friends. Eddie quickly responds, *No guts, no glory.* Seve texts back, *Is my trailer still there?*

For the next hour I ease my way around the vast, glistening lake and find a motel in South Tahoe. The smell of pine is strong. Asking where I might get a decent meal, I fall into conversation with Claudio—he's in his mid-twenties and from Romania. He came to work for the summer season but stayed on.

"People here are more smiling," he tells me. "More open. I had to get used to it. Back home people have a wall up. Everyone's face is so serious always. But there's nothing to be sad about all the time in life. You can smile some of the time." Claudio tells me all this with a dour expression. Tall and skinny, his wool hat pulled down low, his eyes are dark, with dark circles below them.

"You ever get lonely so far from home?"

"Of course," Claudio says, as if stating the obvious. "But I like the people here more. Easier to make friends."

"And what's the most important quality in those friends?" I ask, as I so often have across America.

"Loyalty," Claudio announces without hesitation. "Not talking bad behind your back." It's the single attribute that has proven the most important among nearly every one of the younger men I've spoken to on the topic.

When night falls, I walk across the street and back into Nevada and enter Harveys casino. The place is quiet, between seasons, the summer crowd gone, the skiers not yet arrived. There's one roulette table open. It's empty, and I pull out my five dollars.

"Hundred-dollar buy-in," the croupier tells me.

"Oh, I just want to play one number." My voice is plaintive.

The tiny Asian woman behind the table looks around, then jerks her head in a go-on-hurry-up gesture. She scoops up the silver ball and flings it around the wheel.

I place my chip.

"Good luck." She nods.

I watch the ball zip at unnatural speed, the numbers spin.

When the croupier sees where I've placed my bet, she glances up at the board indicating the ten most recent winning numbers. "Look," she says, and I follow her gaze. The number at the top is 35 black.

"Oh," I say. Had this been the start of my trip back in Atlantic City, I might have attached metaphorical significance to this— "I'm too late. I've missed my opportunity. My friendships have come and gone." But having crossed the country and experienced them all again, I know that is not the case. They are there, and strong, in some ways stronger than ever for the passing of time and the efforts made—their value understood in a way it could never have been in youth.

"That's my number." I shrug to the croupier.

"Never know," she says brightly.

We watch. The ball drops down among the spinning red and black squares and begins to bounce, the wheel slows, the silver ball settles—21.

"We try," the croupier chirps, shrugging.

"Someday," I call over my shoulder and walk back into the night.

The following morning I'm having a carelessly prepared and overpriced breakfast at a café in something called the Shops at Heavenly Village, just off the main drag in South Tahoe. It's the kind of soulless, upscale outdoor mall that could be placed almost anywhere where there is money. Simon and Garfunkel's "Homeward Bound" is being piped throughout the compound, and it feels suddenly very much like my accidental exploration across America is drawing to a close.

Today the early sun will slash through the pines on Route 89 as I climb out of town. Route 88 will take me over Kit Carson Pass and through Eldorado National Forest. I'll skirt alpine lakes and see bald, snowcapped peaks with views across the Sierra Nevada range—one more gasp-inducing experience of America—until the road descends through golden rolling grasslands of the Central Valley. I'll detour slightly into Lodi in order to blare the old Creedence Clearwater Revival song of the same name (*Oh, Lord, I'm stuck in Lodi again!*) as I cruise through town. Then it will be all multilane highways and interstates to San Francisco Bay and my rendezvous with Don.

Berkeley, California

Standing on the stoop outside my hotel, it occurs to me that one of the obvious ironies on this trip of reconnection of 9,759 miles has been the extraordinary amount of time I've spent alone. But in a very real way I was never alone. The spaces in between have been filled with an America that has offered itself up to me—people who surprised me in their unguardedness, their accessibility and generosity, their willingness to hold out a hand to one of their own passing through.

I've cruised byways that were desolate and remote, and narrowly escaped harm on truck-choked interstates. I've chased ghosts in Appalachia and Texas, and ran from them in Kentucky and Nevada.

From one side of the country to the other I've encountered men whose friendships have lasted for decades upon decades—friendships that are so close that neither can imagine life without the other. I've met men who have no male friends at all, who can't even conceive of the idea. I've met men who yearn for deeper connection, and those who have found it in men's groups. I've met young men who readily admit to their loneliness and older men who deny it. I saw and experienced the solace offered by camaraderie, repeatedly and freely offered up.

Then a white, well-worn SUV comes rolling up, right on time. Don's genial face breaks into a wide grin from behind the wheel as he flings an arm out the window to wave his greeting. He then climbs out, embraces me, and we head over to one of Don's old haunts, an upscale farm-to-table place with an effortless Northern California charm that takes a lot of work to achieve. Don's been traveling, as he nearly always is. Egypt, Japan, the Galapagos, Paris, Japan again.

"My little guy, Rowan, is dying to go to Japan," I say.

"We'll take him!" Don gushes. Few people communicate with as many exclamation marks as Don.

The very quality that first drew Don and me close is the thing that might have kept us distant—and what has kept numerous other acquaintances of mine confined to a cordial level. I came into the field of writing, and travel writing specifically—which Don had pursued with great success for decades—from the perceived grander and more public platform of show business. That some met me with quiet resentment was something I understood and accepted—I kept my head down and went to work. But instead of leading with any complicated feelings he might have felt, Don met me with a bemused amiability. And it's something we discuss for the first time over dinner.

"I was confident in my own value," Don says simply. Consequently, mild pangs of jealousy over whatever added attention I received amused him about himself and held no sway over him. He was able to own his reactive feelings, his humanness, with detachment and the same curiosity with which he viewed me. Meanwhile, I could perceive Don's self-awareness, and more than that, I could sense the innate generosity that sprang from him. We met in that area of understanding, and in so doing, forged a quick and lasting mutual trust.

"Trust is a word I've heard again and again on this trip," I say. "What's the one word that comes to mind for you when describing friendship?" I ask Don.

"Understanding," Don says. "You?"

"Safety."

"That makes sense, given what we were just talking about, coming from the show biz world you do, and people projecting all kinds of things."

Don and my conversations tend to be deceptive in their depth, since we laugh so much—or maybe it's the laughing that allows candor, doubts and fears, dreams and aspirations to slide out so unguardedly. It is a definition of friendship that such intimacies can be readily shared with a person one sees so infrequently.

When Don's wife had a serious health scare a few years ago, he emailed a cluster of friends, asking for prayers and "good vibes."

"Not everyone would do that," I say.

"I'm not afraid to ask for help," Don says simply.

"A lot of men are."

"Well, I love people."

"I won't hold that against you, but what I'm saying is that in writing an email like that, by letting your friends in, you're admitting to a kind of vulnerability, and a lot of guys wouldn't. They'd say that if they were to admit that vulnerability, it would make them seem weak. And that's one of the near-universal things I encountered across the country—the desire among men to not appear weak."

"Well, that's just stupid." Don laughs.

"Emotionally articulate as always, Don."

"What do you expect? I'm a writer." He laughs again. It's a loud, full-bodied, and unembarrassed laugh. It's a laugh that makes those around him laugh as well. Then, turning serious, Don asks, "What else did you find?"

"One of the deepest and most consistent undercurrents I found across the country, from cowboys, musicians, sensitive guys, tough guys, was the sense that, as men, we feel the weight of providing, of taking care of and being responsible for our people. And that can feel isolating."

Don considers the point. "I feel this. I don't talk about it or even think about it overtly or explicitly much at all, but when you mention it in this way, yes, I share that sensation. I know that my family members could definitely provide for themselves without me, but at the same time I feel that it's fundamentally my responsibility to take care of them. No one has ever said this explicitly to me, and no one has ever asked me to do this. It just feels like a responsibility that I've assumed.

"Now that my kids are grown and out of the house and well along on their own careers, I don't feel this on the same surface level that I used to—it's a much, much deeper sensation in regard to them now, but still, if for some unexpected reason they ever needed me, I'd of course be there."

The following morning we're driving past cypress trees, bent crooked by the years and winds. We're climbing through the Marin mist on our way to Muir Woods and its grove of redwoods. "A walk through the giant sequoias seems like an appropriate way to complete a trip across America," Don suggested at dinner the night before. We park, and the rain feels like it is coming from all sides.

"This isn't rain," Don enthuses. "It's just fog."

"Stop being so fucking ebullient, Don."

We wander along Redwood Creek, straining our necks, gawking, then through the giants of Cathedral Grove and make our way up Fern Creek Trail. We come to two divergent paths and debate which to take. "You ever been lost?" I ask. "I mean really lost?"

Don considers. "No, I don't think so."

"Me either," I say. "It's good to remember that. But I think it would be a good thing to have experienced."

"Emotionally lost is another story." Don's robust laugh echoes through the tall trees.

"What makes you so happy, Don?" I'm not even sure I'm asking a serious question. But Don offers a considered answer.

"I learned a long time ago not to sweat the small stuff."

I regard my friend. "What else?"

His answers come easily. "Tell the people in your life what you want to tell them. Figure out what you want to do and do it wholeheartedly. Say yes to yourself. And when faced with a decision, ask, 'What will make me happy?'"

Don's answers read like platitudes, yet coming from a friend who I know has actively chosen to live a happy life, their simplicity resonates.

"Just don't start hugging a tree, Don."

Don has a prior commitment in the afternoon and so after agreeing to meet again for dinner, he drops me at his favorite café. "I wrote my Lonely Planet book about how to be a travel writer in this café. In that booth." Don points to a table in the corner in the back of Caffè Strada, on the corner of College Avenue and Bancroft Way in Berkeley. Outside, there are dozens of built-in benches and tables on a large patio under fruit trees.

Directly across the street from the college campus, it's a haven and meeting place for students.

Settling down under a pear tree on the patio with a cup of too-strong tea, I check in on Seve. He surprises me by announcing he's breaking down cardboard boxes. I tell him I'll be coming down sometime in the next month. "So you can look forward to that with fear or in loving anticipation," I tell him, laughing.

"It'll be both." Seve laughs louder. "It'll be both." When I do head down to Baltimore two months later, I'll discover he's well along in retaking control of his apartment.

While I'm finishing a second cup of tea on the patio, my phone rings. It's a female acquaintance calling to ask for an introduction to someone I know. I mention I've been out on the road reconnecting with some old friends. Her reply is immediate and direct—"Well, that's good. 'Cause guys have no idea how to nurture a friendship."

My many conversations across the country seem to bear out what numerous studies show—that male friendship is in steep decline. More and more, men are navigating the world without the support of friends. Loneliness abounds. And people left isolated have increased instances of poor physical and mental health. And conclusions drawn in the isolation of one mind alone can lead a person wildly, dangerously astray.

But why are we men seemingly so bad—and getting worse—at friendship? Is it, as Lew and Bobby said back in Ohio, fear of judgment or rejection, of being perceived as weak? Shame, like Derek and Joe pointed out in Sedona, certainly comes into play. And we are not helped by an inability or unwillingness to communicate.

But I saw signs of hope. Very few of the men I talked with on this trip had ever spoken about the topic of their male friends or analyzed their experiences with male friendship. And while some were initially hesitant, and a few remained guarded throughout, not a single man I asked declined to speak with me about the topic. The vast majority, after their initial surprise, were game to jump in and kick the idea around. A great many opened up and discovered things about themselves and their own views on friendship they weren't aware they held. And most men prolonged our conversation even as I was ready to wrap it up, even the more guarded and defensive men. "I've just never talked about this before," I heard often. "This is actually really interesting to talk about" was another common remark.

I've been brought closer to my friends on this trip—by seeing them again, of course, but even more so by the fact of actively acknowledging our friendships. Like so many of the men I met along the way, we had never previously talked about the value or import of our relationships. In doing so we took greater responsibility for our connection, confirming ownership of our bond in a way that we hadn't before. From those discussions an added generosity resulted, coupled with deeper affection. We feel known by the other to a degree that we weren't before—the words spoken rooting our goodwill and solidifying the commitment to our bond.

A simple comment made to me half a country ago, during my conversation with Larry and Steve back in Austin, Texas, has stayed with me. "Friendship," Larry said, "isn't something intense. It's normal."

This trip has been a revelation on the value of that "normal." These reunions have helped to not only arrest and reverse my growing trend toward a self-imposed isolation, but done so playfully, joyfully, and easily. Nothing could be more ordinary—more normal—than laughing with my friend, sharing my anxieties, listening to his. I needed to do little besides show up. The simple paradox is that other than the ridiculous amount of driving I've done, there is no big deal in what happened these past weeks with Seve and Matthew and Eddie and John and Don, and with all the men I've met who've been generous enough to talk with me and wrestle with the topic of friendship in their lives.

The rewards of my cross-country efforts far outweighed the discomforts of the road or any emotional risk I at times felt. These reunions have helped me to reclaim access to an expansive, secure, playful, and generous part of myself I thought had been worn down by life, or at the very least, a part I felt I could no longer readily access. How grateful I am to have been proven wrong.

We men so often hold ourselves to some imagined ideal—an ideal that simple connection supersedes and proves unnecessary, even false. Back while driving in Kentucky, talking on the phone with Seve, I quoted Joseph Conrad's panoptic truth from *Lord Jim*—"Nobody, nobody is good enough." Yet with the accompaniment of friends—friends to hear us, to receive us, friends to understand and forgive us, to trust and accept us with grace and compassion, to laugh with us, to travel alongside us toward our better selves—we are capable of being much, much more than good enough.

Don and I share another dinner of laughs and candid conversation. After, we head the few blocks back over to Café Strada for a final coffee. We find one of the few available benches under a pear tree on the large patio filled with students—maybe a hundred or so. The fog has lifted. The night is clear, the air milder than it should be for so late in autumn. Occasionally a slight breeze blows. Back in New York it snowed today. I'm sipping a hot chocolate. Don is drinking something called a Strada Bianca Mocha—the house specialty.

Many of the students around us have laptops open on their tables. A few are focused with headphones blocking out the noise around them, but most are gossiping, sipping drinks, laughing, tablehopping—study having yielded to community.

Don and I watch it all from the distance of years. "You know," Don says finally, "I've reached the point in life where everyone looks vaguely familiar."

We laugh, and our chat drifts idly now, sliding from one topic to the next without agenda. We mention the Dalai Lama, shoes, trees, pretty girls and how invisible to them we've become. We talk UFOs, Samuel Beckett. Our chat is inconsequential—other than in that most important way—friends enjoying friendship.

My phone rings. It's my son Sam. It's three hours later in New York than it is here in California. I answer, because I always answer when one of my kids calls. "You're up late, Sammy," I say by way of greeting.

"It's only one," he says. He's been playing his guitar and is eager to share a lick he's working on. Then before I can stop him, he's expounding on something regarding music theory and twelve-bar blues, something I can't understand. Normally I would give free rein to this kind of rant, glad to hear one of my kids so happy and engaged. But after listening for a minute, I cut him short.

"Sammy," I say. "Can I call you in the morning? I'm with a friend."

"Really?" he says, surprised—apparently, he hadn't considered the possibility. "All right, cool," Sam says. "Later."

I smile and we hang up.

Don and I chat and laugh some more. Then we fall silent.

"Thanks for making the time, Don," I say at last.

"Thanks for making the trip," he says.

We lift our cups and touch brims.

New York, New York
Part 2

Six months later, I'm seated in my usual spot at the kitchen table, a cup of weak tea in hand. The dog is asleep in the corner. My daughter, Willow, is perched on a stool at the counter, playing Fruit Merge on her phone. Sam is stalking around the kitchen discussing what kind of guitar he might bring the next time he walks the Camino de Santiago—the five-hundred-mile trek across Spain.

"If you mention the Camino one more time, I'm going to kill myself," Willow says, not for the first time. She then asks if I can drop her to visit one of her friends tomorrow.

"I'm supposed to head down and see Seve. But if he cancels I will."

"Do you think he'll cancel?"

"Fifty-fifty."

Seve has gotten his living situation fully in order, and due to a slight adjustment, his back is no longer causing him such active pain, although he's still seriously restricted in his movement. But given the projected recovery time and Seve's age and the fact he lives alone, there is new talk of not doing the operation at all. I'm headed down to discuss a "game plan."

My phone rings. It's Matthew.

"Sport!" I shout over the line.

"We're gonna get an 800 number tomorrow," he starts right in. "We'll call that and it'll tell us who to contact and when we can go to the bank to get our millions for the dong."

"Perfect," I say. "I could use it right about now."

"Tell me about it."

"What are you going to do with your cash, Sport?" I ask.

He tells me his plan to fly off to see any baseball game he wants at any time.

"Maybe you should buy a plane," I suggest.

We kick around the drawbacks of aircraft ownership—maintenance and the potential hassles with staffing, then agree that simply chartering one as whim dictates is perhaps the best course of action.

"You know what we should do, Sport?" I say. "We get our piles of money in front of us and sit at our kitchen tables and Face-Time and just count out our money together. Every day."

We find this hysterical. We laugh some more. I confirm I'll be waiting by the phone tomorrow and hang up.

"Dad," Sam says. "I've never heard you talk like that with your friends before. Like you've been doing lately. It's really nice."

I'm tempted to remind him that it was his remark that set my trip from sea to sea in motion in the first place.

"Do you think those Vietnamese dong things are actually going to happen?" Willow asks.

"Of course not."

"Then why are you going on about it?"

"Do you know how many laughs we've gotten out of those dong over the past six months? Worth every penny of the hundred dollars I paid for them."

"Does Matthew think it's gonna happen?"
"Well, he's hopeful."
"Your friend is kind of ridiculous, Dad," Willow says.
"I know."
My daughter then fixes me with a glare that screams, "So..."
I smile, then shrug. "He's my friend."

Acknowledgments

Thanks are insufficient for Suzanne O'Neill. This is the third book in which she's given me enough rope to almost hang myself, then stepped in with insight, clarity, and generosity while being indulgent, patient, and exacting. I'm lucky. I am indebted to three dear friends who endured an early draft of this book and offered invaluable insights—Michael Oates Palmer, Lisa Abend, and Dan Wilhelm. David Kuhn is a rock, and there whenever I look over my shoulder for help. Rachel Anne Cantor is likewise attuned.

The team at Grand Central deserves so much of my gratitude. Thank you, Ben Sevier. Thanks as well to my production editor, Anjuli Johnson. Becky Maines needs to be recognized for her discreet and exacting copyedit. Big shout-out to Liz Connor for her brilliant cover design and Bart Dawson for the interior design, including that pesky map. Kudos to Jimmy Franco (and Gina DiBenedetto) in publicity and Tiffany Porcelli in marketing. And I bend a knee to Morgan Spehar for (gently and insistently) keeping everything on track.

Brian Liebman and Cory Richman are always there, always working, and always ready to talk baseball, thank you! Jill Fritzo PR (Jill, Stephen Fertelmes, and Chloe Corkery) handle a drama-filled job with the least drama of anyone I know—thanks for putting up with me. Likewise Katrina Poulos.

Special thanks must go to Seve, Matthew, Eddie, John, and Don, who opened themselves up to me in trust and love and let me spill some of the beans on our friendships. And to all the men who allowed a stranger to approach them and discuss what at times felt like an almost taboo topic, my deepest gratitude.

And then there are Sam, Willow, and Rowan, who continue to teach me daily how to love. And to Dolores, who has taught me more about friendship than anyone (and who still can't ((fu*king)) believe that I, of all people, would write a book about friends).

Notes

BALTIMORE, MARYLAND Part 2
1. Rick Hellman, "How to Make Friends? Study Reveals How Many Hours It Takes," KU News, University of Kansas, March 28, 2018, https://news.ku.edu/news/article/2018/03/06/study-reveals-number-hours-it-takes-make-friend.

ELKINS, WEST VIRGINIA
1. Laura Newberry, "More Than 1 in 7 Men Have No Close Friends. The Way We Socialize Boys Is to Blame," *Los Angeles Times*, October 10, 2023, https://www.latimes.com/lifestyle/newsletter/2023-10-10/more-than-1-in-7-men-have-no-close-friends-the-way-we-socialize-boys-is-to-blame-group-therapy.
2. Daniel A. Cox, "The State of American Friendship: Change, Challenges and Loss," Survey Center on American Life, June 8, 2021, https://www.americansurveycenter.org/research/the-state-of-american-friendship-change-challenges-and-loss/.
3. Ibid.
4. Aria Bendix, "A Stark Social Divide," NBC News, August 25, 2024, https://www.nbcnews.com/health/health-news/close-friendship-social-divide-college-degree-rcna167865#.
5. Maria Vultaggio, "Gen Z Is Lonely," Statista, February 4, 2020, https://www.statista.com/chart/20713/lonlieness-america/#:~:text=Z%20Is%20Lonely-,Mental%20Health,issues%20showing%20up%20for%20individuals%20...
6. Jade Guarnara et al., "The Impact of Loneliness and Social Isolation on Cognitive Aging: A Narrative Review," *Journal of Alzheimer's Disease Reports* 7 no. 1 (June 29, 2023): 699–714, https://pmc.ncbi.nlm.nih.gov/articles/PMC10357115/#:~:text=Additionally%2C%20a%20meta%2Danalysis%20of,or%20social%20isolation%20%5B31%5D.
7. "Loneliness Has Same Risk as Smoking for Heart Disease," Harvard Health Publishing, June 16, 2016, https://www.health.harvard.edu/staying-healthy/loneliness-has-same-risk-as-smoking-for-heart-disease.
8. Michele M. Kroll, "Prolonged Social Isolation and Loneliness are Equivalent to Smoking 15 Cigarettes a Day," University of New Hampshire Extension (blog), May 2, 2022, https://extension.unh.edu/blog/2022/05/prolonged-social-isolation-loneliness-are-equivalent-smoking-15-cigarettes-day.
9. Nancy Schimelpfening, "Differences in Suicide Among Men and Women," Verywell Mind, November 12, 2024, https://www.verywellmind.com/gender-differences-in-suicide-methods-1067508.

10. Dr. Vivek H. Murthy, "Our Epidemic of Loneliness and Isolation 2023," US Department of Health and Human Services, https://www.hhs.gov/sites/default/files/surgeon-general-social-connection-advisory.pdf.
11. Emily Katz, "Three Lessons from Aristotle on Friendship," the conversation.com, May 17, 2023, https://theconversation.com/three-lessons-from-aristotle-on-friendship-200520.

POINT PLEASANT, WEST VIRGINIA
1. Adam Gostick, "Harvard Researcher Reveals #1 Key to Living Longer and Happier," Forbes.com, August 15, 2023, https://www.forbes.com/sites/adriangostick/2023/08/15/harvard-research-reveals-the-1-key-to-living-longer-and-happier/.

PIKEVILLE, KENTUCKY
1. "Clay City, Kentucky," World Population Review, 2025, https://worldpopulationreview.com/us-cities/kentucky/clay-city.
2. Joanna Cheek, "Casual Social Contacts Can Help Combat Loneliness and Improve Well-Being During Pandemic, Psychologists Say," CBC News, December 27, 2020, https://www.cbc.ca/news/world/casual-social-contacts-can-help-combat-loneliness-and-improve-well-being-during-pandemic-psychologists-say-1.5852956#:~:text=World-,Casual%20social%20contacts%20can%20help%20combat%20loneliness%20and%20improve%20well,deadly%20consequences%20has%20emerged%3A%20loneliness.

CLARKSDALE, MISSISSIPPI
1. "Rosedale, MS," Data USA, 2023, https://datausa.io/profile/geo/rosedale-ms/.

UVALDE, TEXAS
1. Dalton Huey, "Social Media 'Friend' Describes School Shooter," KXAN.com, May 13, 2022, https://www.kxan.com/news/texas/uvalde-school-shooting/social-media-friend-describes-uvalde-school-shooter/.
2. Eric Levenson, Isabelle Chapman, Andy Rose, and Shimon Prokupecz, "Uvalde Shooter Was a Loner...," CNN, May 22, 2022, https://www.cnn.com/2022/05/25/us/uvalde-texas-school-shooting-salvador-ramos.

MARFA, TEXAS
1. Bianca Di Julio, Liz Hamel, Cailey Muñana, and Mollyann Brodie, "Loneliness and Social Isolation in the United States, the United Kingdom, and Japan: An International Survey," KFF, August 30, 2018, https://www.kff.org/report-section/loneliness-and-social-isolation-in-the-united-states-the-united-kingdom-and-japan-an-international-survey-section-1/.
2. Murthy, "Our Epidemic of Loneliness and Isolation."
3. Department for Digital, Culture, Media & Sport, Office for Civil Society, and Baroness Barran MBE, "Joint Message from the UK and Japan Loneliness Ministers," Gov.uk, June 16, 2021, https://www.gov.uk/government/news/joint-message-from-the-uk-and-japanese-loneliness-ministers#:~:text=SAKAMOTO%20tetsushi%2

C%20Minister%20for%20Loneliness,Civil%20Society%20and%20Loneliness%2C%20UK.

4. "WHO Launches Commission to Foster Social Connection," World Health Organization, November 15, 2023, https://www.who.int/news/item/15-11-2023-who-launches-commission-to-foster-social-connection.

About the Author

Andrew McCarthy is the author of four books, *Walking with Sam*, *Brat: An '80s Story*, *Just Fly Away*, and *The Longest Way Home*—all *New York Times* bestsellers. He is an award-winning travel writer and served for a dozen years as an editor-at-large at *National Geographic Traveler* magazine. Andrew has directed scores of television shows; his recent documentary, *Brats*, debuted at number one on Hulu. He is perhaps best known as an actor for the past four decades, appearing in such iconic films as *Pretty in Pink* and *Less Than Zero*. He lives in New York.